WALL PILATES
WORKOUTS FOR WOMEN
SPECIAL MENOPAUSE

From 10 to 15 min Routines for Women for all ages

80 REAL VIDEOS PERFORMED BY A QUALIFIED FITNESS INSTRUCTOR +150 PHOTOS

Easy Exercises and Lessons

28-Day Plan

4-training Programs to Improve Strength, Balance, Flexibility and Lose Weight

MIRA WEBSTER

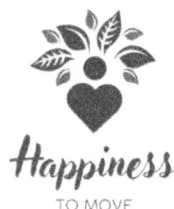

Happiness
TO MOVE

DISCLAIMER

The information contained in this book is solely intended for informational and educational purposes, with the sole intent of providing general information to assist you in your pursuit of physical and emotional well-being. It does not substitute for professional medical advice, diagnosis, or treatment. Before beginning any fitness program or making changes to an existing one, seek the advice of your physician or another qualified healthcare provider.

The author and the publisher of this book are not responsible for any injuries or health issues that may arise from the use of the information contained in this book.

HAPPINESS TO MOVE

My name is Mira Webster and I have been a certified fitness instructor since 2010. From a young age, I have been involved in sports and physical activities. Initially, I participated in team sports like volleyball and field hockey. Later, I dabbled in karate for a while before transitioning to regular gym workouts.

At the age of twenty, I fell in love with swimming, which I still practice today. When I turned 24, I began studying Latin American dances. In 2009, I discovered Zumba Fitness, which completely captivated me. Starting in 2010, I obtained various fitness certifications and credentials, launching my career as a fitness instructor.

My classes are designed for adults and seniors, both using body weight and incorporating equipment such as chairs, steps, dumbbells, Pilates balls, resistance bands, and more. For over 13 years, along with my husband, who is also a fitness instructor, I have been bringing the "joy of movement" to my students

TABLE OF CONTENTS

GET YOUR FREE GIFT

DOWNLOAD YOUR VIDEO WORKOUT PLANS AND THE OTHERS BONUS BOOKS

Finally, you can follow day by day your lessons of

"WALL PILATES WORKOUTS FOR WOMEN" 4 TRAININGS PROGRAMS VIDEOCOURSES.

Practicing your 28-day wall Pilates workout has never been easier. Go to the last page, scan the QR code and gain instant access to:

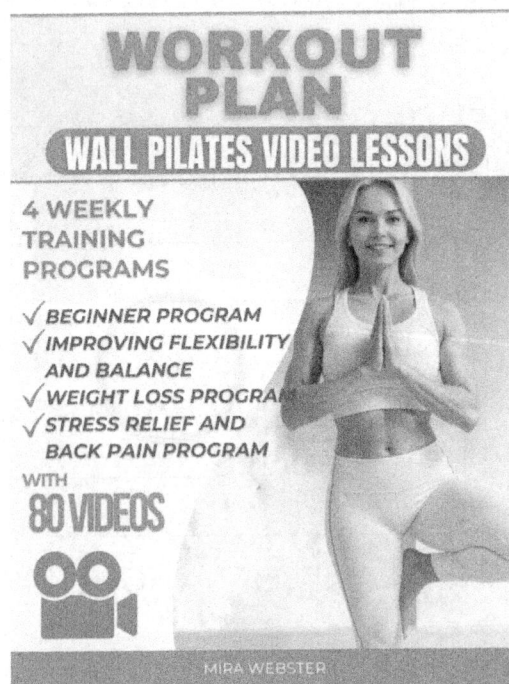

- **WALL PILATES VIDEO WORKOUTS PLAN** -4 weekly programs, featuring 25 video lessons performed by a qualified fitness instructor;

1. INTRODUCTION

Welcome to the world of Wall Pilates! I have created this guide to help you embark on a path to wellness from the ground up, making it suitable for both beginners and older individuals. If you are eager to start on the path to achieving a strong and agile body and mind, one step at a time, this guide is exactly what you've been looking for. In this book, you'll become acquainted with and learn the basic fundamentals of Wall Pilates. I will provide you with the tools to experience the power of this exceptional practice.

Before we dive into this fascinating journey, I present a general introduction to Pilates. This will enable you to understand the basics and appreciate the benefits of this training method that goes far beyond simple exercise.

Ready to learn all about Pilates? Great! Let's get started right away.

What is Pilates?

Pilates is a type of holistic workout where the mind and body are closely connected. The three cornerstone pillars of Pilates are:

1. Breathing,

2. Posture,

3. Control of movements.

The inventor of this method was Joseph Hubertus Pilates, a man who managed to combine Eastern wisdom with the Western approach. In doing so, he created a unique experience that today is embraced all over the world.

It's important to know that in Pilates, **the quality of movement is much more important than the quantity of repetitions**. It's not about performing frantic movements, but about developing a deep awareness of our bodies, learning to feel, listen to, and control our muscles. People trying Pilates for the first time often feel as if they are discovering body parts and muscles they didn't know they had!

If you have never practiced fitness, or if you are transitioning from other types of physical activity, you will be amazed at how Pilates leads to a deep awareness of yourself.

Mindfulness is a key characteristic that Pilates helps you to hone and improve. This addresses not only the physical aspect, but also teaches us to have a deep self-awareness within ourselves."

"What distinguishes Pilates from other types of training? You need to know that in Pilates, and in all disciplines derived from it, the 'core' muscles, often referred to as the 'powerhouse,' are of central importance; indeed, they are the true engines that drive every movement. But there's more: Pilates is an invitation to focus on precision, fluidity, and control of movements. It's not about rushing; it's about creating a harmonious and deep dialogue between mind and body.

Good. After this brief introduction, let's delve a little deeper.

The Pilates method is based on six key concepts that extend far beyond a simple sequence of movements. These principles are fundamental to achieving the best results from each exercise and to making the practice safe and enjoyable. They also aid in moving with grace and balance. Through attention to detail, they simultaneously strengthen, tone, and sculpt the muscles and body. Beautiful, isn't it?

Here are the six basic principles of the Pilates method:

Breathing

Breathing is essential to ensure better oxygenation of the body and to promote blood circulation. Inhaling and exhaling in sync with movements enhances energy and tissue revitalization. However, initially, it may not be easy to coordinate breathing with movements, so it's important to breathe regularly at first. Once you learn to perform the exercise smoothly and naturally, you can then focus more on your breath.

Concentration

Keeping your mind focused on performing the exercises promotes a better muscle response. Being present and aware of the movement and the muscles involved improves control and, consequently, the execution and effectiveness of the exercise.

Control

Every movement in Pilates requires detailed control. This involves being aware of the entire body, from the position of the head and neck to the upper and lower limbs, and including the trunk, back, and abdominals. Although it may seem complicated at first, with practice, it will become automatic within a few days. This will improve the harmony and fluidity of the movements.

Center of Gravity or 'Core'

Also known as the 'powerhouse,' this refers to the muscular area of our body located between the end of the rib cage and the lowest portion of the pelvis; it is the focal point of the Pilates method. Strengthening this area has multiple benefits, which we will explore in detail below. Overall, a strong 'core' promotes correct posture and enables control of the body during exercises.

Precision

Performing exercises with care enhances their usefulness and benefits. Paying attention to detail improves the effectiveness of the exercises and muscle coordination.

Fluidity of Movement

Movements in Pilates are practiced harmoniously and continuously until they become almost elastic. This approach avoids excessive stiffness or movements that are too fast or too slow. Fluidity of movement fosters balance, control, and coordination of movements.

Does it seem too difficult? Don't worry, it will be much easier to do than to describe. It may seem complicated at first, but I assure you that once you start practicing, you will find great satisfaction. **Consistent, step-by-step practice of these key elements will lead you to a greater awareness of your body and mind, and you'll see immediate benefits, both physically and mentally.**

Over the years, Pilates has evolved into many forms, ranging from Pilates MatWork to Pilates using specific equipment like the Reformer for posture and addressing specific health issues.

Did you know that many scholars and teachers have been inspired by Pilates? They have created new, customized methods to meet, in an increasingly attentive and caring way, the needs and goals of their students and clients.

Recently, Wall Pilates has been introduced. It allows for very gentle and gradual body training, without the use of special equipment. All you need is a wall and a mat to lay on the floor.

Are you ready to find out what this is all about? Then continue reading in the next chapter.

2. WHAT IS WALL PILATES

Let's dive into the concept of Wall Pilates. Imagine combining the wisdom of Pilates with the use of a wall for support. This is the essence of Wall Pilates: a method that leverages the stability of the wall to further improve balance, flexibility, and strength. The wall becomes an invaluable ally in the pursuit of correct posture and ideal spinal alignment. Additionally, it provides stable support, enabling even beginners, those who have never exercised, or those who have passed their prime, to train effectively, easily, and safely.

Thus, Wall Pilates becomes a suitable physical activity for most people, especially for those who are new to the Pilates method and are trying it for the first time. Whether you're a beginner or a senior, the wall offers a welcoming presence with kindness and support.

For those starting from scratch on their Pilates journey, **the wall provides stability and security, enabling them to perform the exercises in a more controlled and correct manner**. For older individuals, the wall serves as a bulwark against the passage of time, a reliable benchmark to keep their bodies active and vital for a long time.

You might be wondering now: what makes wall Pilates so special? At first glance, it might not seem obvious, but in reality, the wall helps you develop greater awareness of your body and posture.

It invites you to experience movement in a new way, and simultaneously, it can aid in improving flexibility and strengthening the body's deep muscles. The wall then becomes a support, a reference point, a trusted friend that guides you in performing each exercise.

Moreover, the factor of **balance** should not be overlooked. With the support of the wall, many exercises can be performed more safely. This is particularly advantageous for older individuals, as balance tends to decline with age. Wall Pilates allows you to work on balance gradually and comfortably. Consequently, as time and years pass, you will be able to maintain energy, strength, and confidence in performing daily activities.

It's not over yet: the wall is not just a physical support, but also a creative stimulus. Performing Pilates exercises with the wall as a reference presents a real opportunity to explore new movements and to learn how to properly align the spine and the entire body.

This is not a feature to be underestimated. It's not uncommon to see even young people with closed, forward-bending, or slightly hunched postures. **Practicing spinal alignment, stretching, and strengthening exercises will allow you to get to know your body in depth and discover how even the smallest adjustments in movement can make a significant difference during practice.**

In essence, Wall Pilates is a practice that welcomes all ages and fitness levels. It is an invitation to connect with your body in a new and exciting way, using the wall as a guide and ally in the exercises. No matter your starting level, Wall Pilates offers you the chance to discover a new world of wellness, flexibility, and vitality.

Are you ready to begin the journey toward a new, stronger, more agile version of yourself? Then get ready to discover the wonderful world of Wall Pilates and make friends with your wall of wellness!

3. PILATES: AN ALLY AS WE AGE

Before we continue on our journey into the world of Wall Pilates, I want to take a moment in this chapter to focus on an aspect that is fundamental to a healthy future and important to be aware of: we will explore aging and how the Pilates method can become a trusted companion in old age.

Aging is a natural stage of life, a journey during which changes occur that involve both the mind and body. As we enter or progress through this stage, our bodies undergo progressive changes that affect internal regulation, adaptation to the environment, and our functional reserves.

Roy J. Shephard, Professor Emeritus of Applied Physiology at the University of Toronto, reminds us that age can be categorized as 'middle-aged,' 'elderly,' 'very old,' and 'long-lived.' However, it is important to remember that everyone has their own personal journey, and it can vary greatly from individual to individual.

The body, marked by the passage of time, undergoes transformations that can affect various systems, especially the muscular and skeletal systems. However, the respiratory, cardiac, brain and nervous, immune, endocrine systems, and metabolism are not immune to changes either.

What are these changes and transformations?

In our muscle system, for example, muscle fibers undergo changes such as a slowdown in the pumping of calcium ions and a reduction in mitochondria, our energy centers. This results in a lower metabolic capacity and reduced muscle strength.

The phenomenon known as sarcopenia, which involves the loss of muscle mass, can contribute to motor disabilities and a decline in metabolism.

In the skeletal system, the loss of bone mass increases the risk of fractures, while tendons become less elastic and more fragile.

Overall, the musculoskeletal system may be weakened, limiting the ability to move and function on a daily basis.

Reduction in muscle strength and muscle power is a hallmark of aging.

Decreased muscle strength and bone density are among the first signs of aging, which also affect the overall functioning of the body. The other changes associated with aging are as follows:

- Respiratory capacity decreases, leading to greater fatigue;

- the cardiac system may pump blood less effectively, potentially resulting in heart disease or stroke;

- the brain and nervous system gradually become less responsive, leading to a progressive cognitive deficit, which over time may manifest in daily actions or in the development of neurodegenerative diseases;

- the immune system may weaken, meaning the body can become sick more easily;

- the endocrine system may become less efficient in the production and management of hormones, so hormonal imbalances are common;

- the basal metabolic rate slows down, therefore insulin levels in the blood rise, potentially leading to increases in weight and fat mass.

Now, let's delve into the heart of Wall Pilates in old age. This practice proves to be a valuable ally in maintaining a balance between body and mind, addressing tension and poor posture. This holistic approach works on various aspects:

Breathing: Through conscious breathing, Wall Pilates improves respiratory function and oxygenates the body.

Relaxation: Muscle, mental, and environmental relaxation help reduce tension and promote a sense of well-being.

Mobility: Targeted exercises in Wall Pilates increase joint flexibility and muscle strength, allowing for greater agility in movement.

Balance: Specific exercises enhance the ability to maintain vertical balance, improving stability.

Psychomotor Mastery: By improving coordination and mastery of one's body in movements, one can face daily challenges with greater confidence.

The Wall Pilates method offers a comprehensive experience that can improve and maintain motor skills during the aging process.

Moreover, like all regular and consistent motor activity, this method also aims to slow down the physical and mental aging process.

As you may have gathered from reading this far, Wall Pilates in old age is more than just a physical practice. It is an opportunity to maintain an active body and mind, facing aging with grit and confidence.

Wall Pilates, regardless of your age, is the key to achieving complete well-being. It is an invitation to face and live through the passing years with vitality and wisdom.

4. UNDERSTANDING MENOPAUSE: BIOLOGICAL CHANGES

To better understand the **changes that accompany menopause**, it is useful to explore the biological modifications that occur during this period.

As menopause approaches, the **ovaries undergo slow, gradual, and profound changes**. During a woman's fertile life, the ovaries produce one egg per month and large amounts of **estrogen** and **progesterone**. However, with the onset of menopause, the follicle-rich ovarian tissue begins to transform into stroma, an interstitial connective tissue that produces less estrogen and more androgen. This stroma is the "glue" that keeps the eggs in place during youth, and in the second stage of life, it becomes more connective tissue-rich and egg-poor.

Normally, each month, one of the ovaries produces an egg while the other rests, as if the ovaries were coordinating with each other. From the ages of 35-40 until full menopause, women go through a period known as **perimenopause**. During this phase, sex hormone levels progressively decrease, menstrual cycles become shorter and increasingly without egg production. This leads to **lower progesterone production**, resulting in a relative excess of estrogen.

This **hormonal imbalance causes several symptoms**. The first sign of advancing menopause is an increase in follicle-stimulating hormone (FSH). The quantity and quality of menstrual flow change, becoming irregular. The mucosa lining the uterus (endometrium), stressed by the increase in estrogen not balanced by progesterone, becomes more fragile, prone to bleeding, and thickening of the uterine walls.

During this period, many women experience symptoms such as **breast tightness, mood changes, water retention, exhaustion, malaise, and headache**. Female well-being depends on maintaining a delicate balance, in which progesterone plays a key role.

As the years progress, **estrogen levels also begin to decline**, leading to irregular menstrual cycles (**premenopause**) until menstruation ceases completely, marking the beginning of **menopause** proper. The hypothalamus and pituitary gland continue to send stimulus signals to the ovaries, increasing FSH and LH levels, but the ovaries respond less and less to these signals.

During climacteric, estrogen production by the ovaries does not cease altogether, but decreases significantly. Other organs, such as the adrenal glands, partially compensate for this decrease by producing steroids such as androstenedione and testosterone, which are then converted to estrone (a form of estrogen) in adipose tissue and muscle by an enzyme called aromatase.

These **biological and hormonal changes explain many of the symptoms and changes that women experience during menopause**.

With a clear understanding of these processes, it is possible to better cope with this transitional period with appropriate coping strategies aimed at overall well-being.

5. UNDERSTANDING MENOPAUSE: AN OVERVIEW OF HORMONAL CHANGES

During menopause, a woman's body goes through a series of hormonal changes that can vary significantly from person to person. These changes depend on factors such as physical constitution, fat deposits, and muscle mass. This variability explains why some women experience more severe symptoms than others. For example, women who undergo surgical removal of the ovaries lose endogenous hormone production and therefore may experience more intense menopausal symptoms.

Contrary to what some pseudoscientific theories suggest, the ovaries do not atrophy completely during menopause. In fact, while the volume of the ovaries decreases, especially in the cortical part where the follicles mature, the inner part continues to produce hormone-acting substances that are crucial to a woman's overall and sexual health. The adrenal glands play an important role in this hormonal balance by synthesizing androstenedione, which is then converted into estrone, the predominant form of estrogen during menopause.

Progesterone, although in minute amounts, is also produced by the adrenal glands in both men and women, as it is a precursor to many adrenal hormones.

In the menstrual cycle, estrogen dominates in the first phase, while progesterone, produced by the corpus luteum, dominates in the second phase.

Estrogen stores energy from food in adipose tissue, while progesterone helps turn this fat into energy.

An **imbalance** between these two hormones can lead to disorders such as **fluid retention and weight gain**.

In recent years, there has been an increase in conditions such as ovarian cysts, endometriosis, uterine fibroids, and cancers of the female reproductive system. These problems are often related to the loss of hormonal balance. **Chemicals in foods and plasticizers, which act as hormone disruptors or amplifiers, can also contribute to these conditions.**

A significant aspect of modern society is the tendency to treat menopause as an estrogen deficiency disease, similar to the way diabetes is treated as an insulin deficiency.

In the 1960s, the pharmaceutical industry, through gynecologist Robert Wilson and his book "Feminine Forever," introduced the idea that menopause was a condition to be treated with estrogen replacement therapy. This approach led to an increase in female cancers due to overstimulation of estrogen-sensitive organs.

To mitigate these risks, synthetic progesterone was added to hormone replacement therapy, intending to protect the uterus from estrogen overstimulation and cancer risk. However, even with this expedient, the hormones used to treat menopause still cannot be considered completely safe.

Recently, a new category of hormonal substances called SERMs (selective estrogen receptor modulators) has been introduced. Although these have shown a higher incidence of vascular thrombotic phenomena and a limited effect on hot flashes, their long-term efficacy and safety have yet to be evaluated.

As you may have gathered from reading this far, **menopause is a natural phase of a woman's life that involves a series of complex hormonal changes. It is important to take an informed and balanced approach**, considering both the benefits and risks of hormone therapies, and always seek the advice of qualified health professionals.

6. SYMPTOMS AND THEIR CORRELATIONS

During the period before menopause, known as **perimenopause**, many women experience a number of peculiar symptoms.

One of the most common is **menstrual irregularity**. Over time, menstrual cycles tend to shorten, often occurring every 24 to 25 days, with increased menstrual flow.

These cycles can also be ovulation-free, leading to a **decrease in progesterone and a**

relative increase in estrogen.

This hormonal imbalance makes the uterine lining more fragile, causing more frequent bleeding.

Another common symptom is **hot flashes**, characterized by brief, intense sensations of heat rising from the chest toward the face, accompanied by sweating, tachycardia, and sometimes restlessness. These flashes are caused by an alteration in the body's thermoregulatory system and are often related to an increase in luteinizing hormone (LH). After the disappearance of the menstrual cycle, some women may continue to experience these flashes for several years, with varying intensity and frequency.

Women who have greater body fat deposition tend to cope better with menopause, as fatty tissue can convert some substances into estrogen. However, **the reduction of supporting connective tissue in the bladder and vagina can lead to urogenital problems**, such as vaginal dryness and urinary incontinence. These changes can make sexual intercourse more painful and lead to increased susceptibility to urinary infections.

Another frequent symptom is **weight gain**, due to the **slowdown in metabolism** and increased androgen secretion, which causes a redistribution of body fat with more masculine characteristics. This period is often accompanied by a general feeling of bloating.

Psychologically, many women experience a state of discomfort, related to feelings of inadequacy and difficulty in coping with changes. This can lead **to irritability, depression, unmotivated crying, and both physical and mental fatigue**. It is crucial that the woman receives appropriate support from her partner and family during this period so that she does not feel alone and overwhelmed by her fears.

It is also important to recognize that not all symptoms need to be treated with medication. Conventional medicine often uses hormone replacement therapy to manage menopausal symptoms, but this can have significant risks. In the 1930s, scientist Russell Marker discovered that sterol from a Mexican plant, yam, could be used to produce natural progesterone. However, the pharmaceutical industry preferred to develop synthetic hormones for reasons of convenience and profit, despite the potential side effects.

In addition, the experience of menopause can vary greatly depending on cultural and lifestyle influences. For example, Japanese and Mayan women often do not experience typical menopausal symptoms, such as hot flashes, but report different symptoms such as joint stiffness and headaches. This suggests that in addition to biological differences, cultural and environmental factors may also influence the experience of menopause.

As you will see as you continue reading this guide, **an active and natural lifestyle, a healthy and balanced diet, and the use of gentle remedies can help women experience menopause in a more peaceful and beneficial way.**

7. WHAT TO DO IN PRACTICE

Have you ever wondered if a healthy lifestyle and good nutrition can really make a difference during menopause? The answer is yes! A healthy approach can help **manage many of the troublesome symptoms of menopause, such as**:

- Hot flashes

- Night sweats

- Vaginal dryness

- Loss of energy

- Decreased sexual desire

- Mood swings

But that's not all: it can also help prevent:

- Osteoporosis

- Keep the heart healthy

- Protect against the risk of cancer

- Reduce joint stiffness

- Control body weight

- Improve mental efficiency

- Slow down the aging process

These are not miracles but **realistic goals that you can achieve with small changes.** Women who adopt a healthy lifestyle face menopause with more energy and serenity, making better use of the body's natural self-healing mechanisms. Menopause can become an opportunity to improve your life and realize dreams long kept in the drawer.

8.1   How to Improve Nutrition During Menopause

The way we eat has changed dramatically in recent centuries. Our ancestors consumed wild grains, fruits, berries, honey, and meat or fish caught while hunting. This hunter-gatherer lifestyle changed with the advent of agriculture about 10,000 years ago, leading to a more varied and stable diet that included milk and dairy products and cooked foods.

In the past 150 years, however, industrialization has introduced major changes to our diet. The **refining** of grains, the heat pressing of oils, the processing of salt and sugar, and the use of chemical additives have made **our foods very different from what our ancestors consumed**. These processes have depleted foods of essential nutrients and introduced substances that our bodies struggle to recognize and metabolize properly.

In recent decades, the situation has worsened with the use of genetically modified organisms (GMOs) and the adulteration of foods.

These changes have altered the balance of gut bacteria, increasing intestinal permeability and causing immune problems such as allergies, asthma, and dermatitis.

How can we improve our nutrition, especially during menopause? The answer may lie in returning to a **more natural diet with more whole and less refined foods**. Dr. Kousmine, for example, suggested that many degenerative diseases are caused by modern industrial techniques that deplete foods of vitamins, minerals, enzymes, and polyunsaturated fatty acids, which are essential for our body's biochemical reactions. He proposed a return to a diet more like that of our ancestors: natural, whole foods free of chemical additives.

8.2 Active Lifestyle

Let us not forget the importance of an **active lifestyle**. A sedentary lifestyle, so common in modern life, contributes significantly to the onset of disease. Incorporating regular physical activity can make a big difference. Walking, yoga, biking, or any other activity you enjoy can help keep your body healthy and better manage menopausal symptoms.

In summary, adopting a **healthy lifestyle and a balanced diet can have a significant impact on managing menopause symptoms and maintaining overall health**. It's not just about preventing or relieving symptoms, but also about improving your quality of life and approaching this phase with energy and positivity. We are here to help you find the right balance and live this period of your life to the fullest.

8.3 Acidification of the Body and Its Consequences

During the menstrual cycle, a woman's body eliminates many accumulated acids. But where do these acids come from? Uric acid comes mainly from animal protein, acetic acid from sweets and fats, oxalic acid from cocoa and spinach, tannic acid from coffee and black tea, and lactic acid from muscle activity. The body has different ways to handle these acids; in the case of women, the monthly flow helps a lot in the disposal of these substances.

When menopause comes and the monthly cycle stops, the body has to find new ways to get rid of the acids. **These acids, if not disposed of, can cause irritation, inflammation, weakening of mucous membranes and blood vessels, accelerating aging and increasing the risk of degenerative diseases.**

To deal with excess acid, the body combines it with minerals taken from its reserves. If these reserves are insufficient, the body resorts to bones and teeth.

The modern diet, rich in animal protein and refined sugars, tends to be very acidifying. In addition, stress and the use of chemical drugs further contribute to the acidification of the body.

After menopause, the female body tends to behave similarly to the male body in terms of eliminating acidic waste. However, while the male body is accustomed to this process, the female body must adapt to new ways of elimination.

During fertile life, women's mineral reserves are less stressed, but after menopause, the body must draw more from these reserves.

If the diet is low in minerals, the body draws from the bones, nails, and hair, causing problems such as hair loss, brittle nails, and osteoporosis.

When acids are still in excess, the body neutralizes them by forming salts that are deposited in predisposed areas such as the hips, buttocks, thighs, and belly. How can we correct this state of affairs?

8.4 How to Improve the Situation

Adopting an alkalizing diet can make a big difference. Here are some practical tips:

1. **Eat alkalizing foods every day**: Consume plenty of **fruits, vegetables, legumes, and oil seeds**. These foods help reduce acidity in the body.

2. **Avoid acidifying foods**: **Limit** your intake of **animal proteins, sweets, and refined grains**, which contribute to acidification.

3. **Drink plenty of water**: Water is essential to help the body **eliminate acidic waste**. Try to drink at least 8 glasses of water a day outside of meals.

4. **Exercise regularly**: Exercise helps eliminate lactic acid produced by muscle activity and keep the **body in balance**.

5. **Stress management**: Relaxation techniques such as **yoga, meditation, and deep breathing** can help reduce stress, which contributes to acidification.

Adopting these changes can help you better manage menopause and improve your overall health. Remember, it is important to listen to your body and make choices that make you feel good.

8. DOWNLOAD SPECIAL IN-DEPTH GUIDE E-BOOK "NUTRITION IN MENOPAUSE" WITH RECIPES

Give your health a boost!

Continue your deep dive into nutrition in menopause by downloading the complete guide of over 150 pages and discover how to rev up your metabolism, lose weight, and say goodbye to all the bothersome symptoms of menopause.

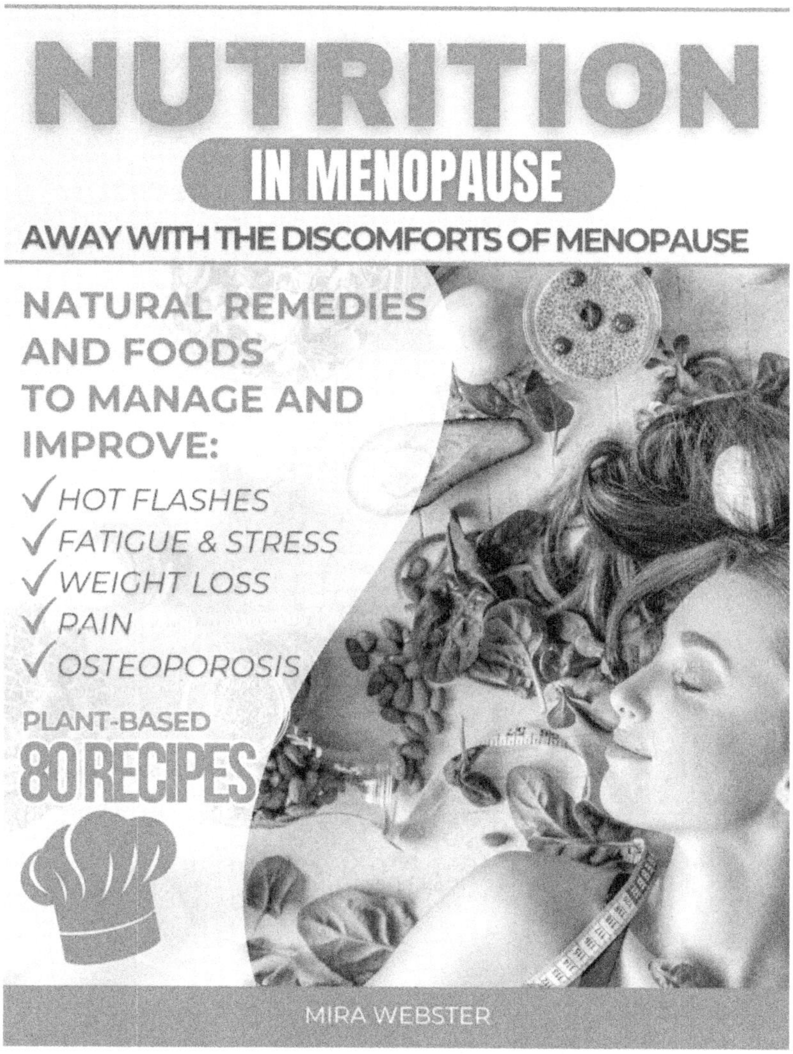

NUTRITION IN MENOPAUSE
AWAY WITH THE DISCOMFORTS OF MENOPAUSE

NATURAL REMEDIES AND FOODS TO MANAGE AND IMPROVE:
✓ HOT FLASHES
✓ FATIGUE & STRESS
✓ WEIGHT LOSS
✓ PAIN
✓ OSTEOPOROSIS

PLANT-BASED
80 RECIPES

MIRA WEBSTER

To download the ebook NUTRITION IN MENOPAUSE now:

1) leave a quick and honest review

2) email me at happinesstomove@gmail.com with subject WP REVIEW DONE

3) I'll reply to you and I send it this beautiful e-book that will help you to:

   a. Understand Menopause: discover all mechanisms that your body activate during perimenopause and menopause

   b. Learn what to do in practice: Discover natural remedies, dietary solutions to bid farewell to the bothersome symptoms of menopause and improve well-being

   c. All about the right nutrition in menopause: learn all macro nutrients, what to eat and what to avoid

   d. 80 plant-based recipes: cold-pressed natural juices, herbal teas, and dishes from breakfast to dessert that are perfect for your menopausal diet.

TO LEAVE A QUICK REVIEW SCAN THE QR CODE OR GO TO THIS LINK
https://2ly.link/1xzHf

9. THE BENEFITS OF WALL PILATES

Regular motor activity brings benefits on many fronts in both physical and mental health. Wall Pilates perfectly combines these two very important aspects to achieve true long-term well-being.

There are four main benefits that Wall Pilates provides, which can be considered the most important in laying the foundation for a healthy lifestyle. Additionally, there is a whole set of other benefits that are equally important and should be considered.

Curious to find out about them? Let's go through them one by one.

1. LOW-IMPACT WORKOUT:

Wall Pilates is a type of training that is gentle on the joints. This makes it suitable for those who have joint problems or injuries and need to be careful not to overload the joints. As a result, the risk of accidents and injuries is significantly lower than in other types of workouts.

2. IMPROVEMENT OF 'CORE' STRENGTH:

Like traditional Pilates, Wall Pilates is an especially effective workout for strengthening the abdominal muscles. The trunk is a critically important part as it is essentially the 'core' of the body. Having a strong trunk means improving posture while also supporting the back and hip muscles, which is crucial in preventing back pain or lower back pain. Numerous recent studies have also shown that a strong trunk allows for better weight bearing during daily activities, consequently preserving the health of the ankles and knees over time.

3. INCREASED MUSCULAR ENDURANCE AND STRENGTH:

Performing Wall Pilates exercises requires control, which is why they are performed at a pace that is neither too slow nor too fast, but in sync with breathing. Executing movements in this manner not only improves muscular endurance from the very first session but also using the wall as additional resistance further enhances the effectiveness of each exercise.

4. INCREASED FLEXIBILITY:

Like traditional Pilates, Wall Pilates is also known for improving flexibility and range of motion. This involves maintaining good mobility in both the upper and lower limbs for a long time. Being flexible helps reduce muscle and joint tension, thus preventing pain in the knees, hips, shoulders, back, wrists, elbows, neck, and legs. Stretching also improves blood circulation and overall physical performance.

10. BENEFITS ON BONES AND JOINTS

The first benefit of Wall Pilates, as a result of the aforementioned factors, is really seen in the bones and joints. How? Let's examine the case histories.

It prevents the onset of osteoporosis and arthritis:

Wall Pilates is a great ally in this regard. These two conditions can become chronic diseases over the years: osteoporosis puts individuals at risk of fractures, and in severe cases, it can take very little to cause a fracture. Arthritis, on the other hand, generally develops in the joints of the wrists, hands, ankles, and feet bilaterally. The main symptoms of arthritis include swelling, joint stiffness, and pain that occurs at any time, especially at rest.

Practicing Wall Pilates regularly keeps all the joints in the body flexible and helps maintain proper bone density levels.

Promotes Better Posture:

Posture is a very important, yet often underestimated factor that can greatly affect everyone's health. Consider common problems like back pain, sciatica, lower back pain, and neck pain, which can originate from poor posture. That's why it's important to take care of your posture as early as possible, preferably starting at a young age. Why? Maintaining good posture can relieve pressure on joints and prevent pain in the vertebrae, keeping them in proper alignment. Wall Pilates, in addition to working on strengthening muscles, contributes significantly to the awareness of correct posture due to the use of the wall. With regular practice, it will become natural to maintain correct posture in all daily activities as well.

Increases Stability and Balance:

Pilates exercises often involve working on unstable surfaces or through movements that require balance. This type of workout can improve joint stability and overall balance, reducing the risk of falls.

Increases Blood Circulation:

Regular practice of Pilates can promote blood circulation, leading to better oxygenation of joint tissues and promoting overall joint health.

Reduces Joint Load:

Pilates exercises are low-impact, meaning they do not exert as much load on the joints as some other types of exercise. As a result, Wall Pilates is particularly beneficial for people with knee and ankle issues, or for those who wish to prevent wear and tear on their joints.

Promotes Spinal Mobility:

Many Wall Pilates movements involve flexion, extension, tilting, and rotation of the spine. This can help maintain spinal mobility and prevent stiffness.

Stimulates Collagen Production:

Did you know that physical activity, including Wall Pilates, can stimulate collagen production in joints and connective tissues? Collagen is essential for the health and integrity of joints, enabling them to stay healthy and youthful for longer.

Relaxes Tense Muscles:

The stretching and relaxation exercises in Pilates can help reduce muscle tension around the joints, improving comfort and mobility.

Reduces Joint Stress:

Pilates emphasizes movement control and fluidity, which reduces excessive mechanical stress on joints during exercise. The result is less wear and tear over time compared to other physical activities, thus better protecting the knees, ankles, wrists, hips, shoulders, etc.

Let me now remind you of an important concept: As with any form of exercise, Wall Pilates practice should be tailored to individual needs. It's always recommended to consult a health professional, your doctor, or a qualified instructor before starting a new exercise program, especially for those who have pre-existing health problems or specific bone and joint conditions. This will help you adapt your exercise program to meet your specific needs. Also, remember to listen to your body during each practice. Try to understand your limitations, and learn to manage them to gradually improve over time.

11. BENEFITS OF WALL PILATES DURING MENOPAUSE

Pilates during the menopausal phase can offer several benefits to women. Menopause is a transitional period in a woman's life during which there is a decrease in estrogen levels, and a range of physical and psychological symptoms can arise.

Here are some of the specific benefits that Pilates can provide during menopause:

Improves Flexibility:

During menopause, many women may experience increased muscle and joint stiffness. Pilates is known for promoting stretching and improving flexibility, which can help maintain joint mobility and prevent tension buildup.

Strengthens the Core:

Decreased estrogen can negatively affect bone density and muscle mass. Wall Pilates, with its focus on strengthening the core and the entire body, can help maintain muscle strength and bone density, reducing the risk of muscle loss and osteoporosis.

Improves Posture:

Did you know that decreasing estrogen can also affect posture due to changes in bone structure? As you may have gathered from reading this guide, Pilates places special emphasis on proper body alignment and posture. Improving posture can not only reduce the risk of muscle and joint pain but can also positively affect your perception of your body image.

Relieves Stress:

Menopause can lead to hormonal fluctuations that contribute to higher levels of stress and anxiety. Wall Pilates incorporates breathing and concentration techniques that can help you reduce stress, resulting in greater mental calm.

Improves Emotional Well-being:

Physical activity, including Wall Pilates, is linked to the release of endorphins, known as 'happiness hormones.' These neurotransmitters can help improve mood and combat any symptoms of depression that may emerge during menopause.

Promotes Circulation:

Through the fluid movements practiced in Wall Pilates, blood circulation can be stimulated. This can be especially beneficial during menopause, when some women experience decreased circulation and a potential risk of cardiovascular problems

Increases Body Awareness:

During menopause, many women may experience changes in body image and self-perception. Wall Pilates encourages increased body awareness, allowing women to reconnect with their bodies in a positive way.

Promotes Healthy Sleep:

Menopause can affect sleep quality. The relaxation practices and breathing techniques of Wall Pilates can help improve sleep quality and address insomnia issues.

12. BENEFITS ON ANXIETY AND STRESS

Did you know that Wall Pilates can offer significant benefits for anxiety and stress management? These benefits come from the combination of controlled movements, mental focus, and mindful breathing typical of Pilates. Let's take a closer look at how Wall Pilates can help alleviate these widespread issues that affect so many people.

Stress Reduction:

Wall Pilates incorporates exercises that require concentration and mental focus. This helps shift attention from a restless, anxious mind to controlled body movement. The mind-body connection promoted by Pilates can then guide you to a state of mental tranquility, reducing stress.

Breathing Techniques:

The coordination of breathing with movement, particularly in certain Wall Pilates exercises and especially at the end of the exercise routine, is a very important factor. Deep, mindful breathing techniques can activate the parasympathetic nervous system, which is responsible for the body's relaxation response. This can help reduce heart rate and blood pressure, inducing a state of calm.

Muscle Relaxation:

The smooth, controlled movements in Wall Pilates improve flexibility and muscle strength. These movements can help release accumulated tension in your muscles due to chronic stress, leading to a state of relaxation. Muscle relaxation can have a positive impact on the perception of your overall well-being.

Increased Self-Awareness:

Wall Pilates encourages you to pay more attention to the balance, alignment, and sensation of your body in space. This leads to increased body awareness. This awareness may help you distract your mind from anxious thought patterns, creating a state of 'presence' in the present moment.

Stimulation of Positive Neurotransmitters:

Exercise, including Wall Pilates, is associated with the production of endorphins and serotonin, known as the 'happy hormones.' Improving your mood has many benefits, including reducing anxiety and dispelling sadness or negative thoughts. As a result, you will experience a greater sense of well-being, which can extend throughout your daily life.

Increased Mental Flexibility:

Practicing Wall Pilates requires an open and flexible mind to adapt to various exercises and movement sequences. This principle can also be applied to anxiety and stress management, helping to develop a more resilient mindset in the face of daily challenges.

Emotional Tension Reduction:

The stretching and relaxation exercises in Pilates can also help release accumulated emotional tension. This allows you to face challenges with greater clarity.

Retreat Moment:

Wall Pilates practice can be considered a time of retreat from daily stress. By focusing on the practice, you can detach yourself from anxious thoughts, creating a space of mental calm.

It is important to note that the benefits of Wall Pilates for anxiety and stress management may vary from person to person. Regularly practicing this physical activity, in combination with other stress management techniques such as meditation and relaxation, can help create a holistic approach to mental well-being. As previously suggested, if you are facing significant anxiety or stress, it is advisable to consult a health professional to customize your approach and maximize the benefits.

13. WEIGHT LOSS BENEFITS

Generally, Pilates, and consequently Wall Pilates, are not primarily known for fat loss but rather for improving strength, flexibility, posture, and muscle tone. However, some exercises can indirectly contribute to the reduction of body fat mass, especially when combined with a balanced diet and an active lifestyle. Here's how Wall Pilates can affect body fat mass:

Increased Metabolism:

The involvement and activation of both large and small muscle groups can increase basal metabolism in the short term. A higher metabolism means the body burns more calories even at rest, potentially contributing to a reduction in body fat mass over the long run.

Muscle Toning:

With Pilates and Wall Pilates, the goal is to strengthen various muscle groups, including the 'core' (abdomen, back, and pelvic muscles). An increase in muscle mass can improve the ratio of lean mass to fat mass, as muscles burn more calories than fat tissue.

Functional Training and Fat Mass Loss:

Pilates and Wall Pilates exercises often involve multi-joint and functional movements. This type of training can increase energy expenditure during exercise, contributing to a potential reduction in body fat over time.

Insulin Sensitivity:

Insulin is a hormone responsible for regulating blood sugar levels. Exercise in general can improve our body's insulin management, which can positively affect carbohydrate and fat metabolism. Better insulin control means more effective body weight management.

Mental Well-Being:

Stress-eating is a common behavior where people seek food to relieve stress. Unfortunately, this behavior can lead to weight gain. As you may have gathered by now, Pilates and Wall Pilates promote relaxation and mental well-being through the mind-body connection and mindful breathing. The endorphin release generated by the workout helps reduce the desire for excessive 'stress-eating.'

Active Lifestyle:

Regular practice of Wall Pilates can encourage a more active lifestyle overall. An increased level of daily physical activity can help better manage your body weight over time.

If you aim to achieve a reduction in body fat mass, I recommend implementing a holistic approach that includes a balance of diet, exercise, sleep, and stress management. Adding to Wall Pilates a combination of cardiovascular training, strength training, balanced nutrition, and an overall healthy lifestyle can effectively lead to fat mass loss.

14. LOW-IMPACT ACTIVITY BENEFITS

Compared to other more intense forms of exercise, Wall Pilates, as a low-impact activity, offers numerous benefits. Here are the most important ones.

Joint Protection:

Using the wall for support during exercises provides stability to the joints, minimizing wear and tear and overload. This is particularly beneficial for those who are looking for a safe yet gentle workout on the joints.

Lower Risk of Injury:

Low-impact exercises like Wall Pilates reduce the risk of injuries related to excessive impact or abrupt movements. It's important to note that these exercises do not involve jumping or the use of weights. This makes this type of training suitable for people with joint problems, pre-existing injuries, or simply for those who want to avoid the risk of injury during exercise.

Improved Flexibility:

Wall Pilates involves stretching and mobilization exercises that help improve the flexibility of joints and muscle tissues without overstretching. Maintaining flexibility as the years go by is a great advantage, as it makes the body less vulnerable to injury and capable of performing daily activities without effort and fatigue, even with advancing age.

Strengthening Support Muscles:

Although low-impact, Wall Pilates works on the supporting muscles, such as the core muscles, which stabilize the spine and joints. This strengthening improves posture and stability.

Improved Balance:

Using the wall for support helps develop balance safely and increases body awareness in space, reducing the risk of falls and improving coordination.

Blood Flow Stimulation:

Low-impact activities stimulate blood flow without putting excessive pressure on the heart and arteries. Improving your cardiovascular health gradually allows you to gain benefits safely. Your heart can remain strong and healthy over time, enabling you to continue many activities even as you age, while keeping feelings of fatigue and exhaustion at bay.

Suitable for Different Ages and Fitness Levels:

Because Wall Pilates is gentle and customizable, it is suitable for a wide range of ages and fitness levels. It is an excellent choice for older adults, beginners, and those recovering from injuries, or anyone looking for a gradual way to start an exercise program.

Continuity in Fitness:

The low-impact nature of Wall Pilates makes it a sustainable option over the long term. People can continue practicing it over time without the risk of excessive fatigue or overload injuries. Simultaneously, they can improve their physical and mental well-being over time.

In conclusion, Wall Pilates is an excellent option for those seeking a low-impact activity that offers a range of health benefits. The combination of controlled movements, core work, and wall support makes it an ideal activity for maintaining a strong, flexible, and healthy body without placing undue stress on the heart, bones, and joints.

15. BENEFITS ON BALANCE

By now, you will have understood how many benefits Wall Pilates can offer if practiced consistently. It's important to know that the benefits on balance are just as significant. Here are some of the balance benefits of Wall Pilates:

Improved Stability:

Using the wall for support, you can perform a variety of exercises involving bilateral or unilateral movements. These exercises allow you to strengthen your stabilizing muscles. This means that you can achieve improved body stability during daily activities, and at the same time, the risk of falls will be reduced.

Control of Movements:

In Wall Pilates, the focus is on the precise control of movements. This approach will help you develop muscle control and body awareness, which are key elements in improving balance.

Increased Coordination:

Many Wall Pilates exercises involve coordinating different parts of the body in a synchronized manner. This type of work allows you to improve coordination and balance as your body learns to move more harmoniously.

Posture Improvement:

Proper posture is essential for good balance. The slow, controlled movements in Wall Pilates help strengthen postural muscles and develop a more upright posture, which in turn contributes to better balance.

Increased Confidence:

As you improve at performing Wall Pilates exercises and develop greater balance, you will also build more confidence in your physical abilities. This confidence often reflects in greater personal assurance in dealing with everyday situations.

Sensory Training:

Wall Pilates exercises often engage the body's sensory system, including the eyes, inner ear, and touch receptors. This helps improve balance through increased awareness of movements and changes in position.

Better Weight Distribution:

Wall Pilates exercises encourage an even distribution of body weight on both sides of the body. This contributes to greater overall stability and balance.

Reduced Risk of Falls:

Last but not least, improved balance through Wall Pilates can significantly reduce the risk of falls, especially for older adults or those with a history of balance issues.

As you may have realized from reading this guide on Wall Pilates so far, there are indeed many benefits that come from consistent and regular practice of this wonderful workout. Now you have no more excuses for delaying the start of your wellness journey!

Are you ready to begin working out?

In the next chapter, we'll look at all the details of how to set up a Wall Pilates workout. You will learn how to train, how often, at what intensity, and how to start your journey safely and effectively.

16. TRAINING

How to train

When deciding to begin a training journey, whatever your goal may be, it is critical to consider some personal factors to understand how to best approach your practice.

I suggest you get a notebook and answer these simple questions, which will help you think through and carefully choose how to begin your training journey:

1. Is this your first time starting a practice, or have you followed other paths before?

2. How long has it been since you last exercised?

3. When you perform your daily activities, do you experience shortness of breath?

If yes, in which activities do you feel it?

4. Do you experience fatigue if you go for a walk or bike ride?

5. Do you have any specific medical conditions that you need to pay attention to?

6. Have you undergone any medical procedures?

7. Have you suffered any injuries in the past?

After answering all these questions, consider talking to your doctor or a specialist. Before you begin any workout, having the support of a specialist or your doctor is very important to personalize your path, and to ensure that you are performing the exercises that are right for you.

This guide provides you with the knowledge and tools to practice low-impact exercises suitable for seniors and beginners.

Although this is an entry-level physical activity, I recommend consulting with your doctor if you have a medical condition or poor mobility. You will be able to discuss with them any exercises to avoid or prefer, depending on your personal health situation.

Before you start exercising, it is important to understand that effective exercise relies on three basic factors:

- **Sequence of exercises to involve all muscle groups;**

- **Frequency of physical activity;**

- **Intensity of the exercises.**

Involvement of all muscle groups: This ensures a full-body workout and thus results in overall physical and mental benefits.

Frequency of exercise: Practicing 20 minutes of physical activity every day is different from practicing for one hour, for example, only one day a week, and it is still different from practicing every other day.

Exercise intensity: Progression from more basic exercises to more challenging ones should be gradual. This allows the muscles to progress and improve safely while avoiding discomfort or injury. Above all, it allows one to build self-esteem, avoiding disappointment from incorrect or overly high expectations.

With these factors in mind, any training program, regardless of the age at which it is practiced, will be effective and yield the expected benefits.

What does it mean to train? The concept of complete training involves 7 factors:

1. Warm-up

2. Aerobic activity

3. Endurance and toning

4. Flexibility

5. Balance

6. Stretching

7. Cooling down

Before beginning to exercise, each of these factors should be considered and customized to achieve the set benefits and goals. It should be noted that each exercise may involve one or more of these factors simultaneously. For example, a flexibility exercise may also affect balance, or a stretching exercise may also develop flexibility. Even performing the same exercise at different intensities can transform it from a simple warm-up exercise to an aerobic one.

1. Warm-up:

It's important to perform warm-ups before any workout. These exercises prepare the muscles for greater exertion, preventing injuries during training such as cramps, muscle tears, lacerations, and the like. Even a simple 10-minute brisk walk can be an effective warm-up to start an entry-level workout.

2. Aerobic Activity (CARDIO):

The goal of these exercises, over time, is to raise the heart rate. The greatest benefits are to the cardiovascular system and in the loss of fat mass.

3. Resistance and Toning:

Resistance exercises help develop muscles and can utilize tools such as elastic bands or weights. In Wall Pilates, even the weight of one's own body is an excellent resistance tool. The benefits include muscle strengthening of the upper and lower limbs and loss of fat mass.

4. Flexibility:

Flexibility exercises aim to increase a person's ability to make wide movements within the limits of joint capabilities, depending on muscle-tendon elasticity as well as joint mobility. The more flexible one becomes, the greater the ease of movement. The benefits are significant: reduced risk of injury, increased flexibility of the spine and muscles, and maintenance of body posture over time.

5. Balance:

Exercises that help improve balance greatly reduce the risk of falls and simultaneously strengthen the body's muscles, as well as train concentration. They are ideal for achieving mental and physical well-being.

6. Stretching:

These exercises aim to stretch or lengthen muscle fibers, preventing the buildup of lactic acid that causes typical post-workout pain. Many strength, flexibility, and balance exercises include elements of stretching, contributing to both muscle lengthening and toning. Additionally, stretching plays a crucial role in preserving the health of tendons and ligaments. As muscle volume increases due to training, there is increased strain on them. Stretching helps restore the proper balance between muscles, ligaments, and tendons, while also safeguarding joint function.

7. Cooling Down:

This phase includes a series of exercises focused on breathing, aimed at gradually returning the heart and muscles to a state of rest, while maximizing the oxygenation of the entire body. It constitutes the final part of the workout.

The Complete Workout

A complete workout that is effective and aims to obtain the greatest amount of benefit possible involves exercises that incorporate all the previously explained factors. The workout plan you will find in this guide provides a specific sequence, where combining flexibility, balance, and toning exercises will allow you to gradually achieve the expected results.

If you are over 60, I advise you to focus on all aspects of training, especially on the following:

- Practice of respiratory and chest exercises to enhance oxygenation.

- Performance of light aerobic exercises, which are useful for managing diabetes and cardiovascular problems, and for promoting the reduction of body fat.

- Practice of simple resistance exercises of medium to long duration, to increase muscle strength.

- Performance of balance exercises, essential for preventing falls

The Importance of the 'Core'

The 'core,' as you may have gathered by now from reading this guide, is precisely the central part of the body that includes the muscles of the trunk, abdominals, hips, back, and lower back. It represents the core of the entire body, being the most crucial muscular region. Therefore, it is also referred to as the 'powerhouse.' A strong and robust 'core' can provide you with long-term well-being and benefits throughout the body. Practicing some simple exercises in your daily routine can effectively strengthen this area.

Developing a strong, stable, and flexible 'core' by practicing easy exercises daily can help you avoid back pain and reduce knee pain if you suffer from it. This is possible since specific 'core' exercises have been shown to improve the distribution of weight on the lower limbs, consequently reducing the occurrence of pain and disease.

Last but not least, training the 'core' means working many muscles simultaneously. This greatly increases calorie consumption, making the activity effective for burning fat and achieving weight loss goals as well.

17. PRACTICAL RECOMMENDATIONS BEFORE YOU START

Practicing a Wall Pilates program for beginners includes a variety of exercises to be performed using the wall for support, whether standing, sitting, or lying on the floor.

In this guide, you will practice different routines that will help you gradually improve your level to achieve the mental and physical well-being results described in the previous chapters.

Choosing the Right Wall

Choose a stable wall that is wide and spacious. Ensure the wall is free of pictures or shelves, and that there is empty space both at the wall and on the adjacent floor where you will perform the exercises. This is to avoid possible accidents caused by accidental collisions with objects that may be too close.

Mat:

Use a mat that has good thickness, as it will provide extra cushioning. It also helps support your spine, joints, and bones during exercises, whether in standing, sitting, or floor positions.

Clothing and Shoes:

Wear clothing made of cotton or breathable technical fabric. You should feel comfortable; movements should be free from 'hindrances' or friction that can be caused by clothing that is too tight or not stretchy enough. Wear sneakers, or even better, Pilates shoes or non-slip socks. It's important to have stability and to wear specific socks that prevent slipping.

Water and Towel:

Make sure you have your water bottle handy and avoid drinking excessively cold water. During your workout, drink often in small sips. Avoid drinking large volumes of water at once, as you may experience stomach bloating and discomfort during your workout. Also, have a towel ready to wipe sweat from your forehead and hands.

Snacks, Snacks, or Main Meals:

Ensure you eat breakfast or a snack at least a couple of hours before starting your workout. This avoids digestive discomfort or feeling sick during your workout; it's important to avoid straining while digestion is in progress.

Balanced Nutrition:

- Try to follow a healthy diet:

- Have a good breakfast, a healthy lunch, a light dinner, and a few snacks throughout the day.

- Prefer fresh and organic foods, proteins, vegetables, whole-grain carbohydrates, and fresh and dried fruits.

- Avoid refined flours, sugars, heavy cheeses, packaged foods, and sugary drinks.

- Consult a nutritionist for a personalized eating plan.

Prepare Yourself Before Proceeding with Your Monthly Exercise Plan:

Take the time to read the workout plan carefully and familiarize yourself with each exercise included. Practice each one two or three times to gain confidence before actually beginning the workout program.

Set Your Own Pace and Listen to Your Body:

When practicing the exercises, avoid rushing and tune in to your body's reactions. Always start with the easier ones and gradually increase the intensity. If certain exercises are too difficult, reduce their intensity. It's important that you feel mild fatigue, but don't overstep your limits. Between exercises, take a couple of minutes to breathe deeply and drink. Also, consider consulting your doctor to tailor the workout to your specific needs.

Breathing:

Wall Pilates involves focusing on breathing during the practice of each exercise. However, initially, this can be difficult as you need to pay attention to the exercise. When you first practice an exercise, do not think about the breath, but breathe naturally, and especially avoid holding your breath apnea-style. As the exercise becomes familiar and more automatic, you can begin to focus on your breathing.

Practice Meditation and Gratitude:

Devote at least 5 minutes daily to meditation. During these times, breathe deeply and slowly, tuning into the sensations in your body. For added benefit, practice meditation sitting up after your workout, or in the morning right after waking up, or lying down before falling asleep.

Example of a Simple Meditation:

Begin by breathing calmly. Focus on your breath, counting slowly to 4 during inhalation and the same during exhalation. If you prefer, you can add soothing background music, such as the sounds of nature, which might include the sound of streams, the sea, or the chirping of birds.

If your mind starts to wander, allow the thoughts to come and then let them go, without forcing yourself to block or push them away. With consistent practice, you will notice that your mind gradually becomes freer, and you will experience a growing sense of peace and relaxation. End your practice by giving thanks for the positive things in your day, such as the food you ate, the people close to you, or even small things like the sun that warmed your face or the rain that nourished the fields.

Rest:

Sleep has the great power to regenerate organ tissues and flush out toxins. Try to get 7 to 8 hours of sleep each night, and if possible, take a short afternoon rest. Your body will thank you!

Is it possible to improve fitness at any age?

It all depends on you. Age is relative, but it's certain that you can always take your fitness to a better level. Are you feeling out of shape and afraid it's too late to start working out? Don't worry, I have good news for you: it is possible to improve at any age.

Okay, you can't take 30 years off your ID card, but if you decide to implement a consistent workout routine, it's certain that you'll feel stronger, more vital, and energetic. You'll be able to continue doing many activities well into your later years.

Common Alignment Mistakes to Avoid

Maintaining proper posture is essential to avoid injuries in Pilates. Below are some tips for achieving proper alignment:

Neutral Spine:

The back should not be excessively curved. Keep your shoulders relaxed, pulled back and down, aligned above your hips, and keep your chest open.

Activating the 'Core':

Every Pilates exercise relies on stabilizing the 'core' muscles. Without proper activation of this area, incorrect postural habits can form, or back injuries can occur. To activate the core, tilt your pelvis slightly and pull your belly button toward your spine. By doing so, you should feel the 'core' muscles contracting.

Aligning the Joints:

When performing exercises that require you to bend your knees, make sure they do not extend past your toes. For example, in the wall squat exercise, the knees should be aligned directly above the ankles. This alignment concept also applies to other joints, such as in the wall plank position, where the shoulders should be aligned directly above the wrists. You will find details like these in the explanation of each exercise.

18. WARM-UP, MOBILITY, AND CARDIO EXERCISES

STANDING ALTERNATE ARM EXTENSION (WARM-UP)

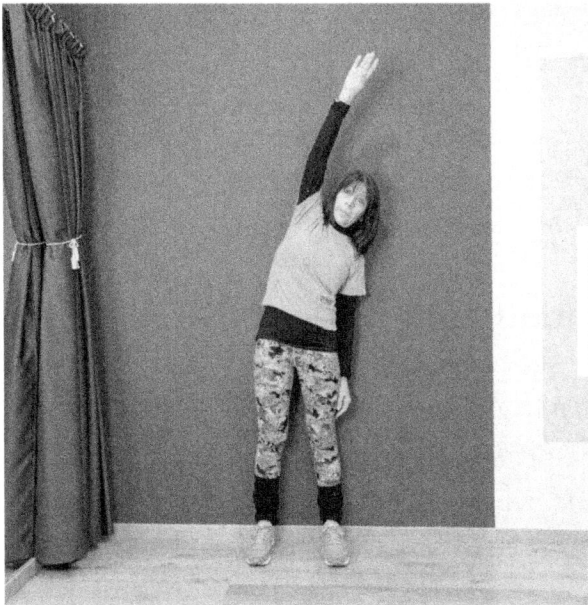

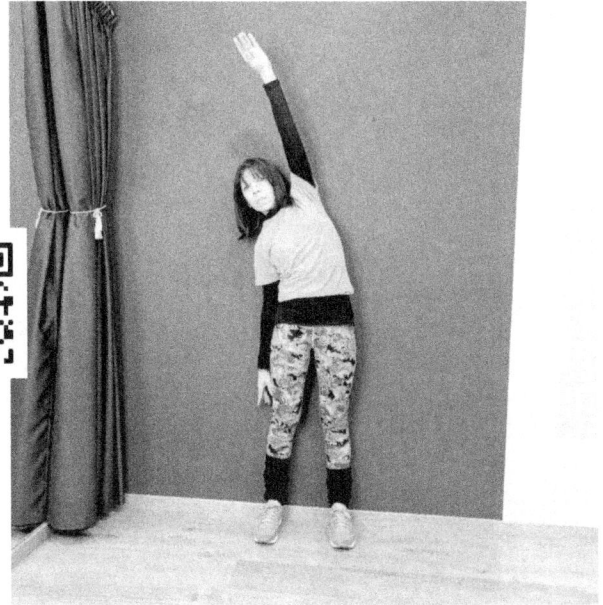

Muscles involved: Stretching of the lats, also known as obliques.

Level: Basic.

Execution: Stand upright with your back resting against the wall. Ensure your head, buttocks, and upper back are well supported against the wall. Place your feet apart at hip width. Keep your arms positioned along your sides. Raise your right arm along the wall, keeping it outstretched, and bring it all the way up over your head, stretching your right hip well. Slowly bring it down and return to the starting position. Repeat with the left arm. Alternate sides for each repetition.

Common Mistakes: Bending the arms, holding the breath, rushing the movement.

Tips: Inhale at the beginning of the movement and exhale as you raise your arm above your head.

STANDING SIDE BENDS (WARM-UP)

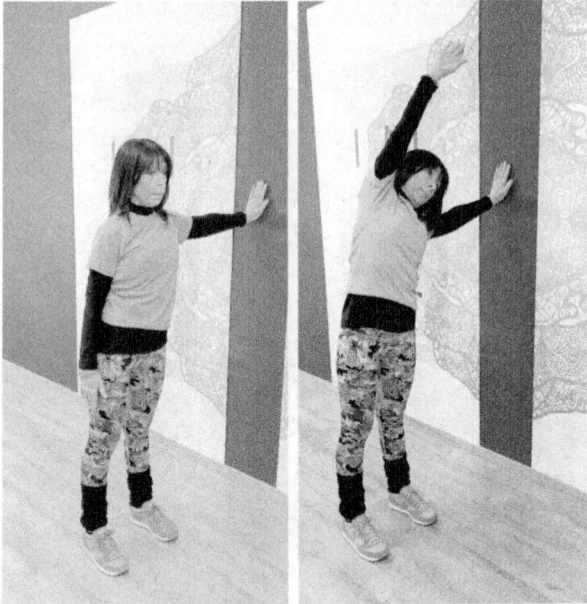

Muscles involved: Stretching of the great spine and oblique abdominals.

Level: Basic.

RIGHT Execution: Stand sideways to the wall. Rest your right hand on the wall, ensuring that your arm is extended. Lean your body toward the right side while raising your left arm up and over your head. Try to make the fingers of your left hand touch the fingers of your right hand. Reach your limit. Return to the starting position.

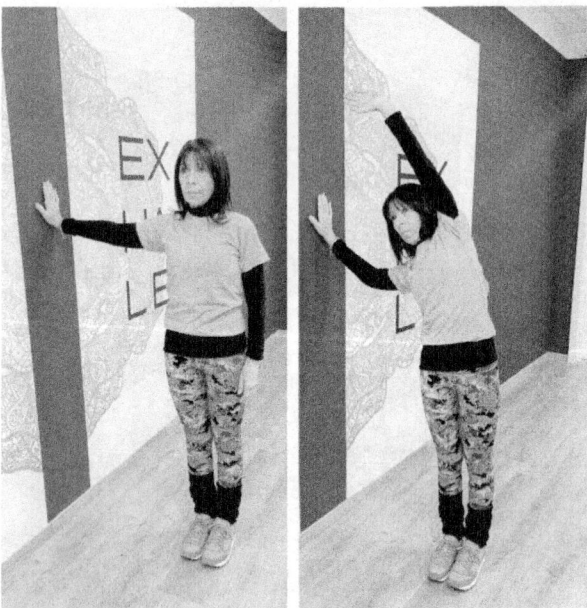

LEFT Execution: Stand sideways to the wall. Rest your left hand on the wall, ensuring that your arm is extended. Lean your body toward the left side while raising your right arm up and over your head. Try to make the fingers of your right hand touch the fingers of your left hand. Reach your limit. Return to the starting position.

Common Mistakes: Bending the arms, bending the legs, arching the lower back.

Tips: If you don't touch the fingers of your hands, it's okay; reach your limit.

STANDING LEG SWING (WARM-UP)

Muscles involved: Exercise that improves hip mobility by dynamically stretching the hip flexor muscles.

Level: Basic.

RIGHT-Side Execution: Stand to the side of the wall. Place your right hand on the wall and your left hand on your hip. From this position, swing your right leg back and forth, keeping your leg straight.

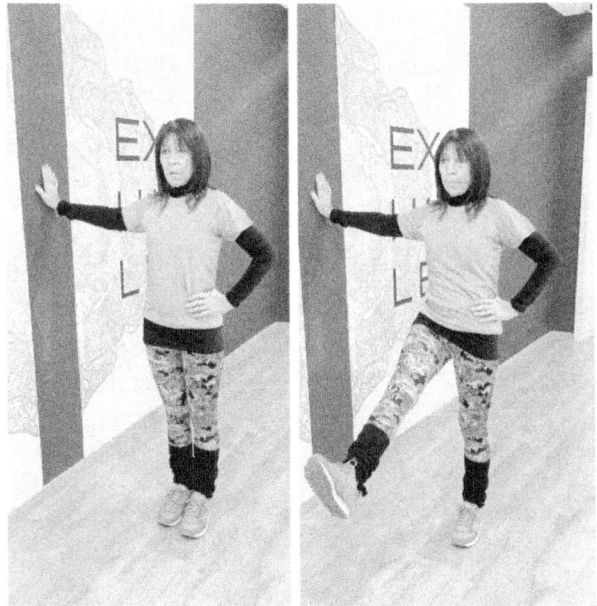

LEFT-Side Execution: Stand to hand on the wall and your right hand on your hip. From this position, swing your left leg back and forth, keeping your leg straight.

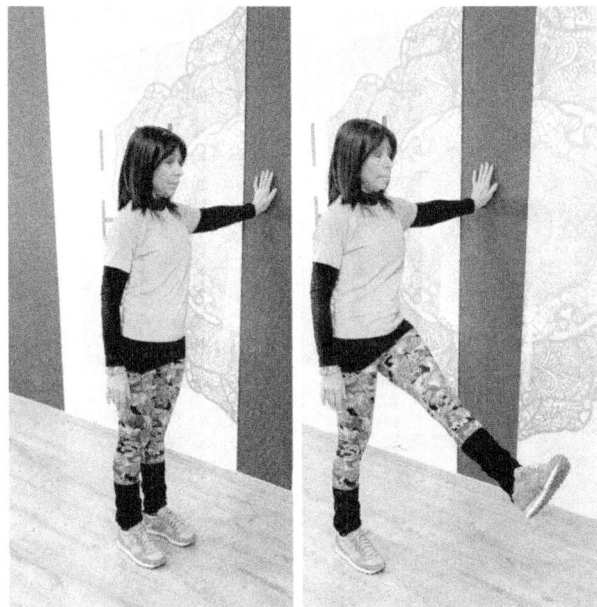

Common Mistakes: Bending your knees, holding your breath.

Tips: Maintain a steady breathing rhythm while performing this exercise.

STANDING LATERAL LEG SWING (WARM-UP)

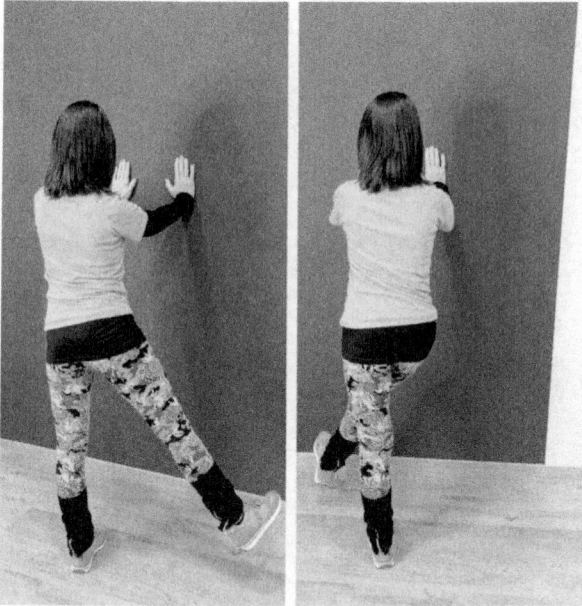

Muscles involved: Hip mobility, dynamically. Great as a warm-up for any leg exercise.

Level: Basic.

RIGHT Execution: Stand facing the wall and place both hands on the wall, keeping your arms extended. Swing your outstretched right leg up to your right side, and then lower it down in front of your left foot. Continue repeating the swing.

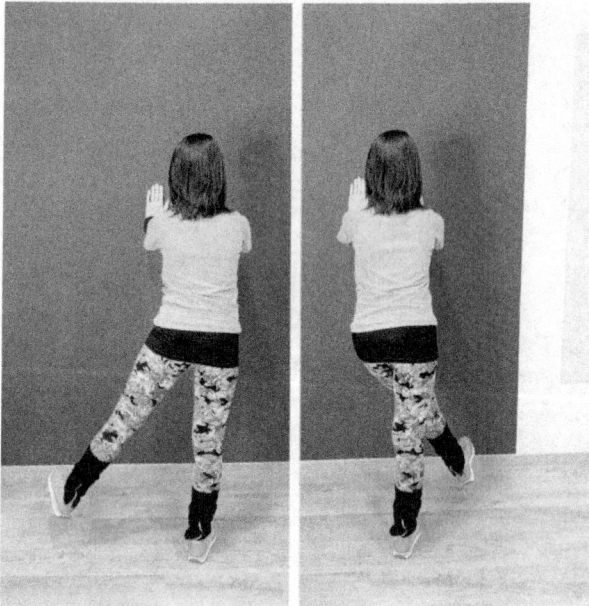

LEFT Execution: Stand facing the wall and place both hands on the wall, keeping your arms extended. Swing your outstretched left leg up to the left side, and then lower it down in front of your right foot. Continue repeating the swing.

Common Mistakes: Bending the knees, holding your breath.

Tips: Maintain a steady breathing rhythm while performing this exercise.

STANDING SIMPLIFIED ANGEL TO THE WALL (WARM-UP, MOBILITY)

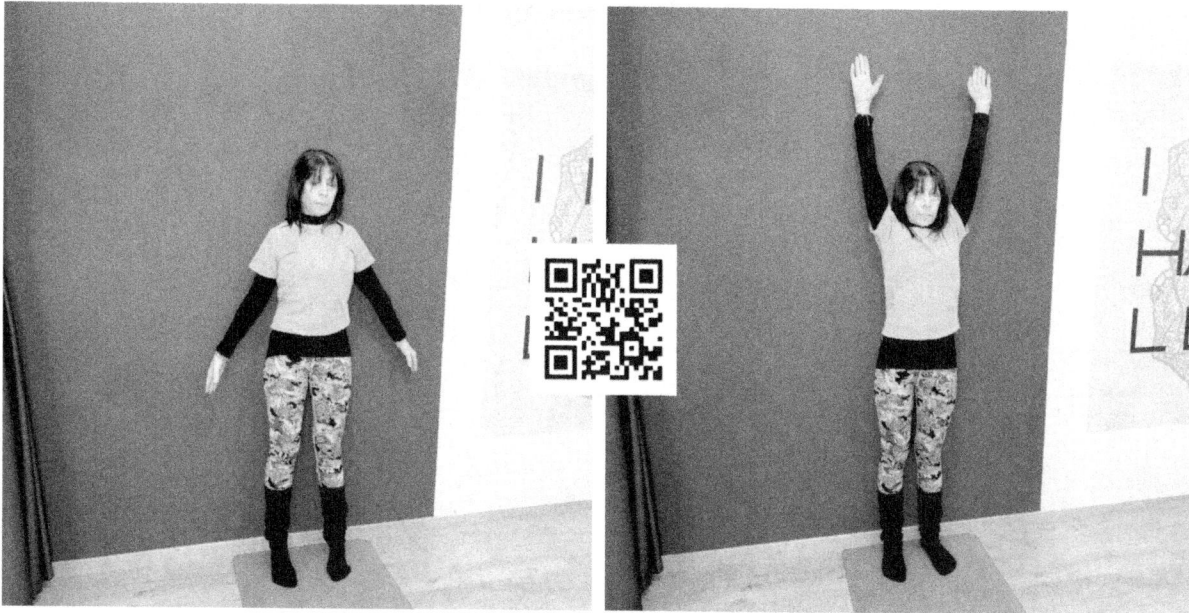

Muscles involved: An exercise that restores posture by activating the muscles of the middle back and improving shoulder mobility.

Level: Basic.

Execution: Stand up straight against the wall. Ensure your head, back, and buttocks touch the wall. Place your hands near your hips. Slide your arms up the wall, raising them toward your head, and reach your limit. When your hands touch, lower them down slowly.

Common Mistakes: Moving too fast, holding your breath, not keeping your back fixed to the wall.

Tips: If you have difficulty keeping your back fixed to the wall, step forward slightly.

STANDING SCAPULAR RETRACTION AND PROTRACTION (WARM-UP, MOBILITY)

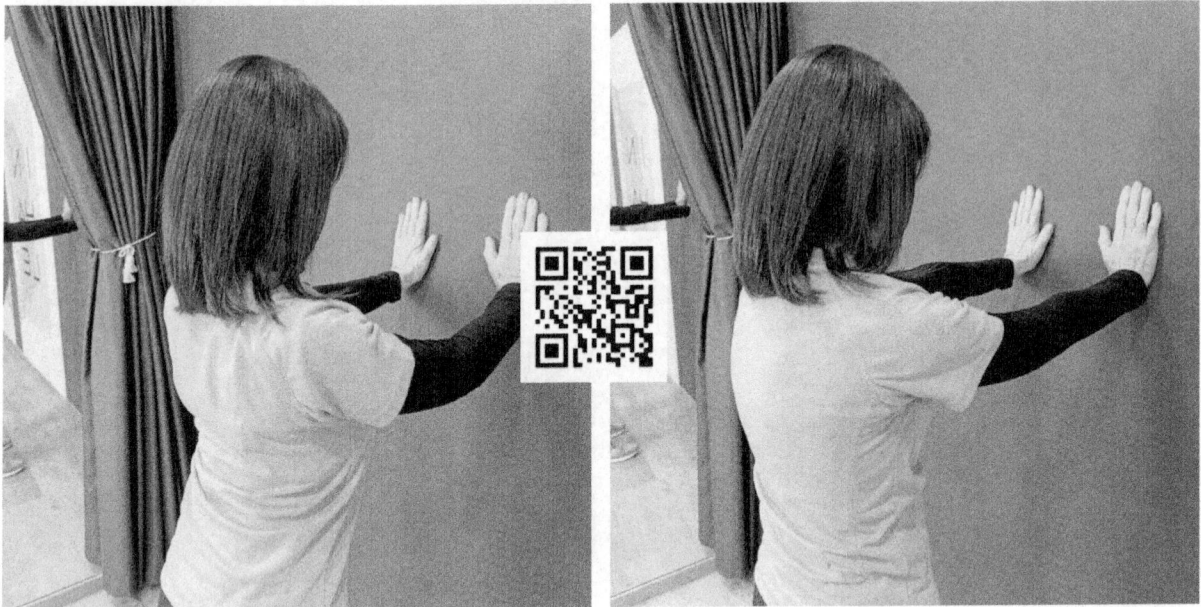

Muscles involved: This is an excellent exercise to activate the muscles of the middle back. It also provides more mobility to the shoulders and stretches the serratus muscles.

Level: Basic.

Execution: Stand upright with feet slightly apart. Place your hands on the wall at chest height, keeping your arms outstretched. From there, slowly bring your shoulder blades together (backward movement). After that, perform the opposite movement, pushing your shoulder blades away (forward movement).

Common Mistakes: Bending the arms, rushing the movement.

Tips: Inhale at the beginning of the movement and exhale slowly as you begin to push against the wall.

STANDING ALTERNATING SHOULDER ROTATION (WARM-UP, MOBILITY)

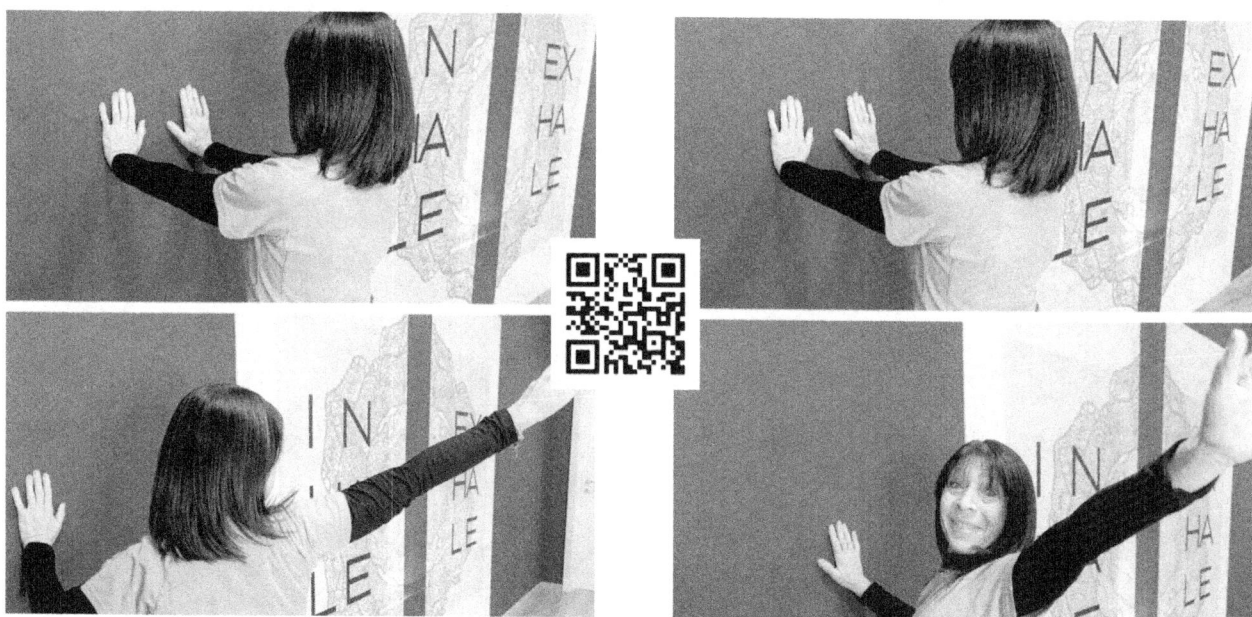

Muscles involved: This exercise is effective for warming up your shoulders before a workout and relaxing them if they are stiff.

Level: Basic.

Execution: Stand upright with your feet shoulder-width apart. Place your hands on the wall, keeping your arms outstretched. Lift and rotate one of your arms backward until you bring your arm behind you to shoulder height (draw a half-circle with your arm). Gently rotate your head toward the rotating arm. Return to the starting position by performing the half-circle in the opposite direction. Switch arms and perform the exercise on the other side.

Common Mistakes: Performing the movement on one side only, bending the arms, going too fast.

Tips: Maintain a consistent breathing pattern while performing this movement.

STANDING ALTERNATING SHOULDER-ARM CIRCLES (WARM-UP, MOBILITY)

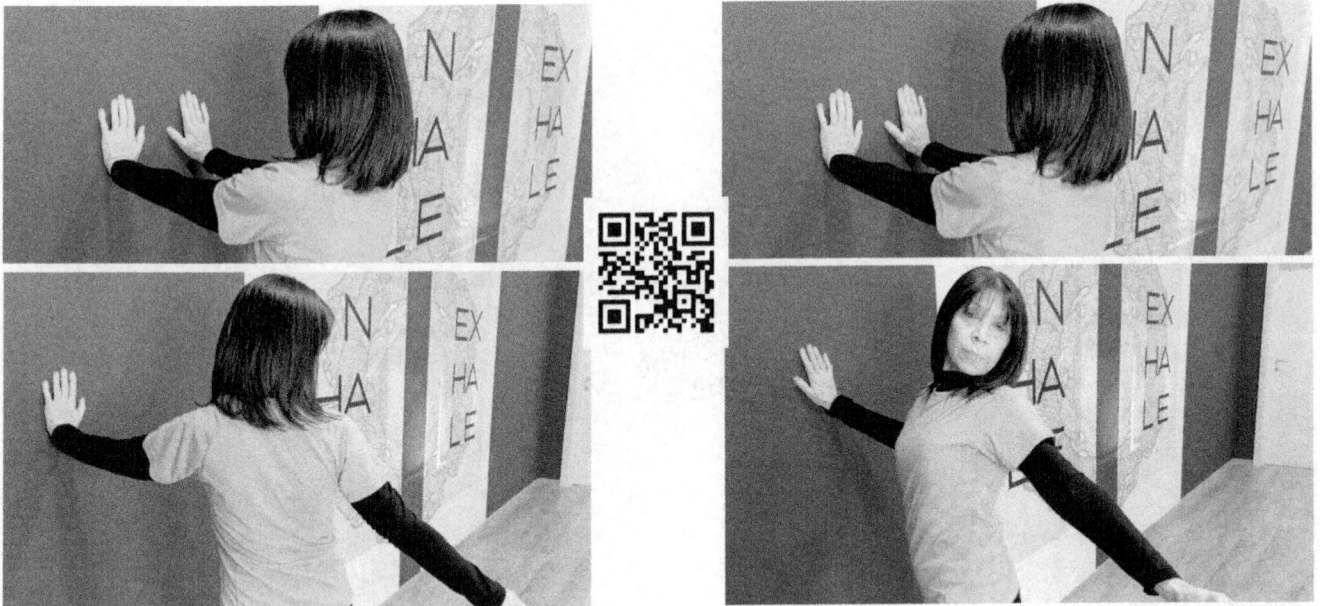

Muscles involved: This exercise is effective for warming up your shoulders before a workout and relaxing them if they are stiff.

Level: Basic.

Execution: Stand upright with your feet shoulder-width apart. Place your hands on the wall, keeping your arms outstretched. Lift and rotate one arm backward, performing a full circle. At the same time, gently rotate your head toward the rotating arm. Perform alternately on both sides.

Common Mistakes: Performing the movement on one side only, bending the arms, going too fast.

Tips: Maintain a consistent breathing pattern while performing this movement.

SEATED ACTIVE FORWARD BENDING (WARM-UP)

Muscles involved: This exercise mobilizes the lower and upper back. It also stretches the hamstrings and calves.

Level: Basic.

Execution: Sit up straight with your back against the wall. Keep your arms at shoulder height and stretch them forward. Keep your legs extended forward. Slowly bend forward until your toes touch your fingers. Slowly come back up.

Common Mistakes: Reducing the range of motion, bending the arms or legs.

Tips: Maintain a consistent breathing pattern while performing this movement.

SEATED KNEES TO CHEST (WARM-UP)

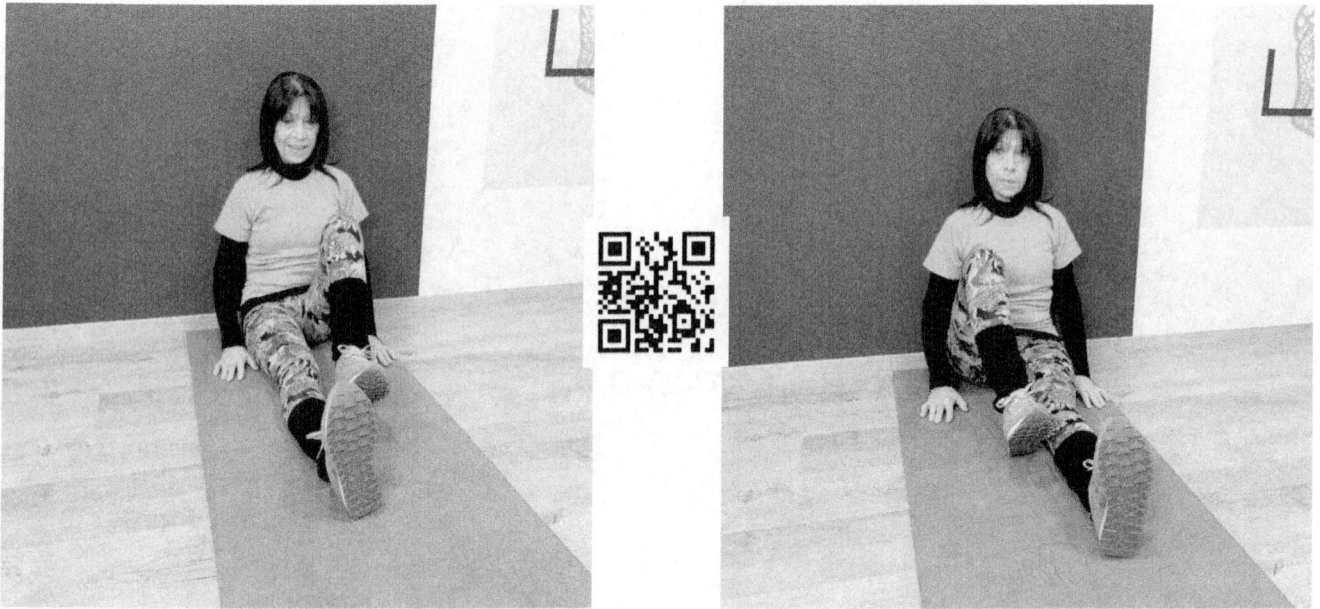

Muscles involved: This exercise activates the hip flexor muscles.

Level: Basic.

Execution: Sit up straight with your back against the wall. Keep your hands close to your hips and your legs extended. Without lifting your heel off the ground, slide one knee toward your chest. Bring it back to the starting position and repeat with the other side.

Common Mistakes: Doing the movement on one side only, bending the lower back.

Tips: Maintain a consistent breathing pattern while performing this movement.

LAY DOWN WALL WALKING (WARM-UP)

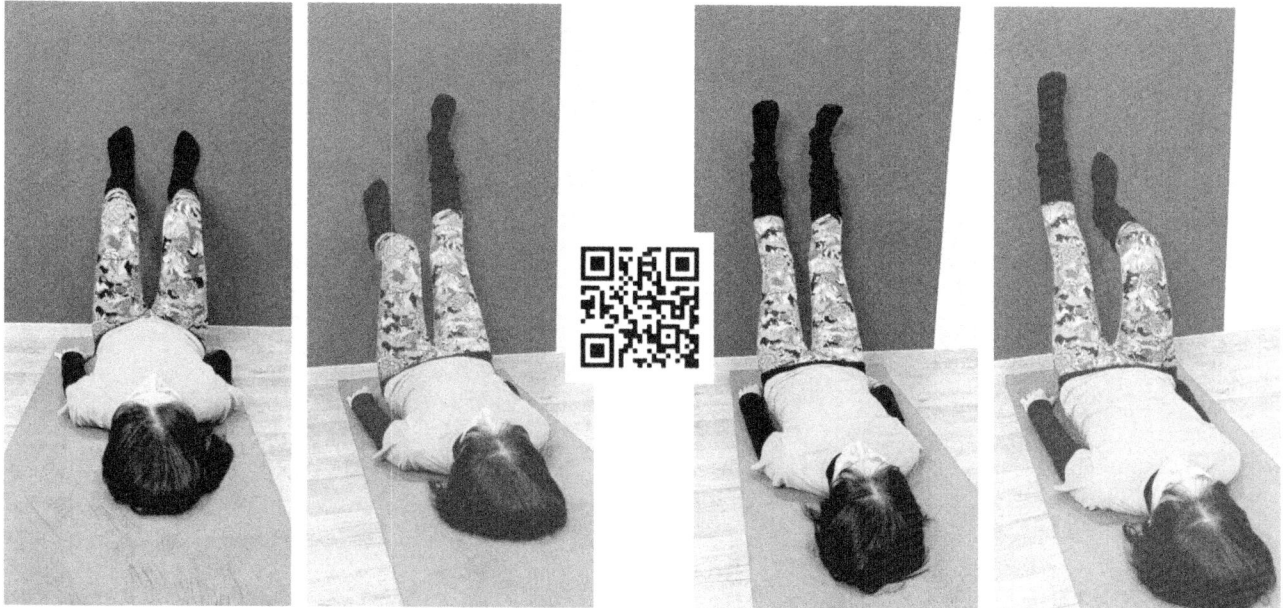

Muscles involved: An easy exercise to start or end a routine. It won't make you fatigued.

Level: Basic.

Execution: Lie on your back on the mat with your knees at a 90-degree angle and your feet resting on the wall. Extend one leg, then the other, then bend the first one and bring it back to the starting position. Do the same with the other. Repeat the exercise from the beginning, simulating the walking motion.

Common Mistakes: Holding your breath, bending the lower back, stretching one leg.

Tips: Keep a consistent breathing pattern while performing this movement.

STANDING CAT AND COW (MOBILITY)

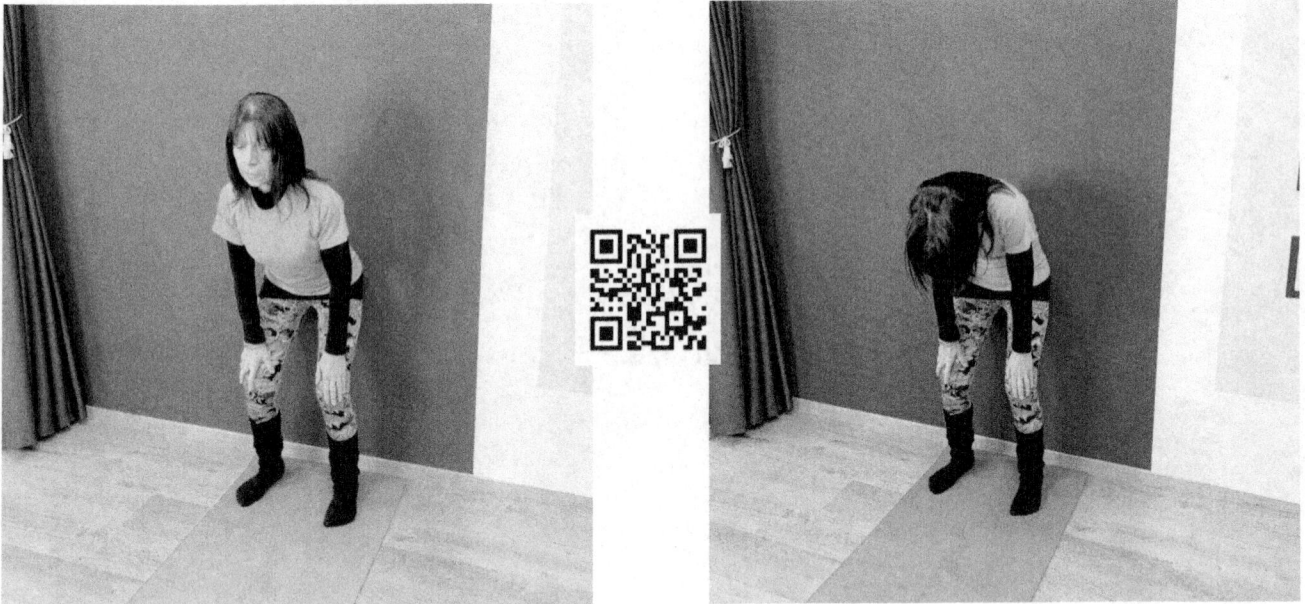

Muscles involved: A fantastic exercise that mobilizes the entire spine.

Level: Intermediate.

Execution: Stand with your back facing the wall. Bend your knees slightly and keep your glutes in contact with the wall. Place your hands on your knees. Arch your spine and gently tilt your head and neck back, then slowly come down a little with your chest. From here, bring your head and neck downward, turn your gaze toward your navel, at the same time bend your spine as cats do and slowly rise back up. Repeat, trying to perform a smooth, continuous movement.

Common Mistakes: Rushing the movement, holding your breath, disengaging the glutes from the wall.

Tips: Inhale at the beginning of the movement as you extend your back and exhale as you begin to bend it.

STANDING CHEST OPENING (MOBILITY)

Muscles involved: A fantastic exercise that mobilizes the entire chest muscles.

Execution: Stand upright with your back against the wall. Your feet are slightly apart at the same width as your hips. Open your arms sideways at shoulder height on the wall. Rotate your palms toward the ceiling. From this position, with your arms extended, bring your hands together, keeping your palms facing the ceiling at all times. Return to the starting position and repeat the exercise.

Common Mistakes: Moving the body away from the wall, holding your breath, going too fast.

Tips: Maintain a regular breathing rhythm.

LAY DOWN HIP MOBILITY (MOBILITY)

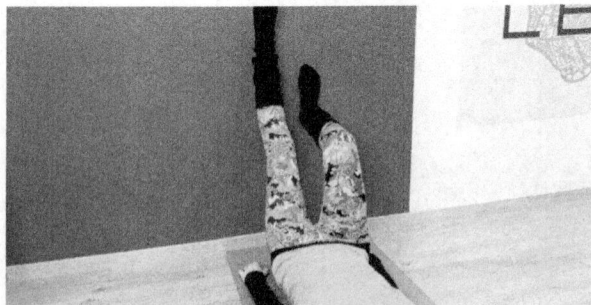

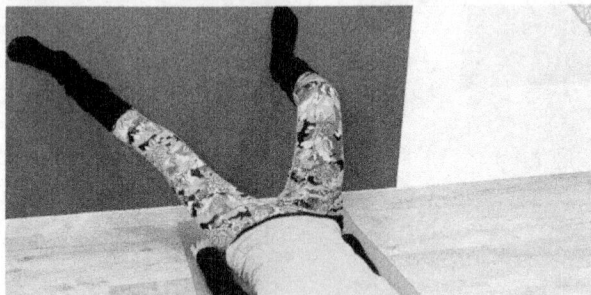

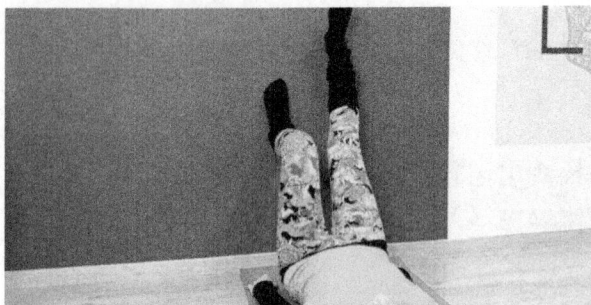

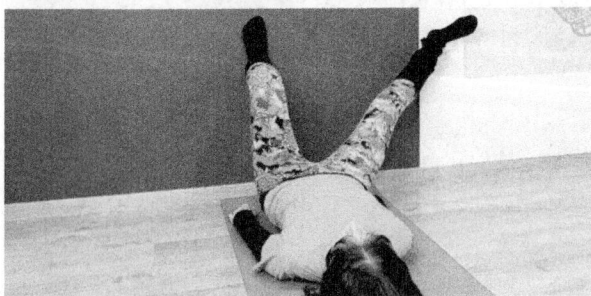

Muscles involved: A fantastic choice for dynamically opening the hips and stretching the adductor muscles. Try it before starting heavier lower body exercises.

Level: Basic.

LEFT Execution: Lie on your back on the mat with your feet on the wall, bending your knees at a 90-degree angle. Extend the left leg and, without moving the pelvis, slide it over the wall on the left side without bending the knee. Return to the starting position and repeat the exercise.

RIGHT Execution: Lie on your back on the mat with your feet on the wall, bending your knees at a 90-degree angle. Extend the right leg and, without moving the pelvis, slide it over the wall on the right side without bending the knee. Return to the starting position and repeat the exercise.

Common Mistakes: Bending the leg, letting the leg fall to the side without control, moving the pelvis.

Tips: Inhale at the beginning of the movement and exhale slowly as you lower the leg.

LAY DOWN ALTERNATE LEG ABDUCTION (MOBILITY)

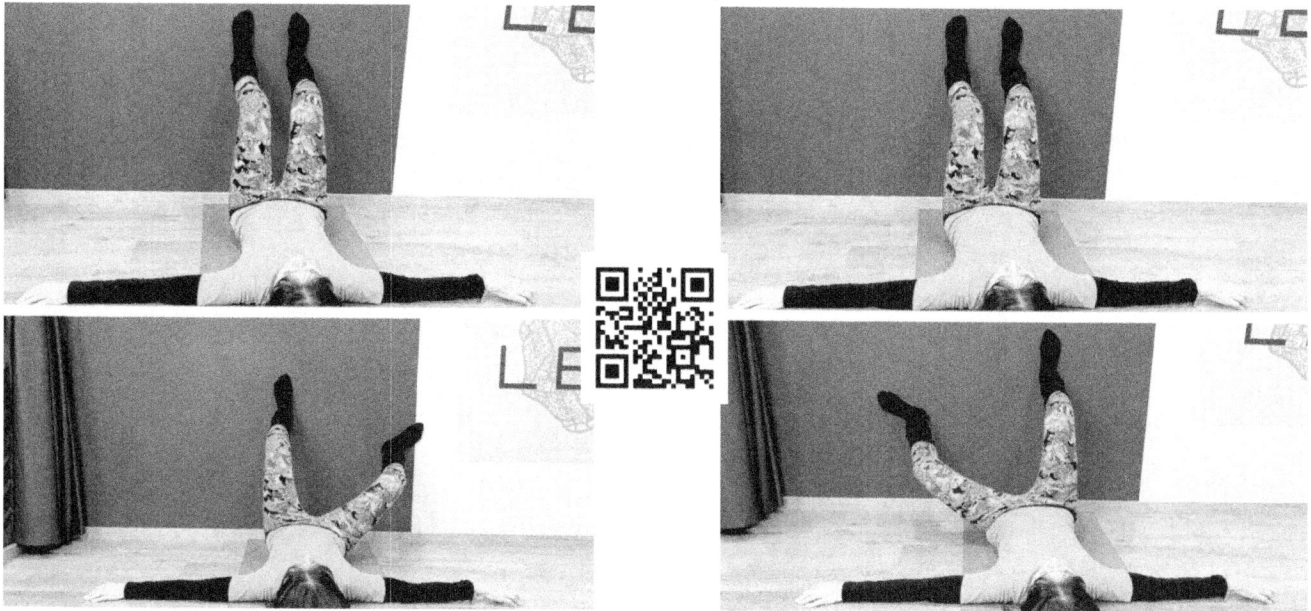

Muscles involved: Alternate leg abduction works on hip mobility and stretches the adductor muscles.

Level: Basic.

Execution: Lie down on the floor with your arms outstretched and open at shoulder height. Place your feet on the wall with your knees at 90 degrees. Slide one foot sideways on the wall while keeping your leg flexed at 90 degrees. Reach your opening limit, then slowly reverse the movement to return to the starting position. Keep your pelvis on the floor the entire time and perform the exercise with the other leg.

Common Mistakes: Bending the lower back, letting the pelvis come off the floor, doing the movement on one side only.

Tips: To keep your pelvis from lifting off the floor, think about pushing your belly button to the floor, then slide your foot to the side.

STANDING KICK-BOX WITH WALL SUPPORT (CARDIO, WARM-UP)

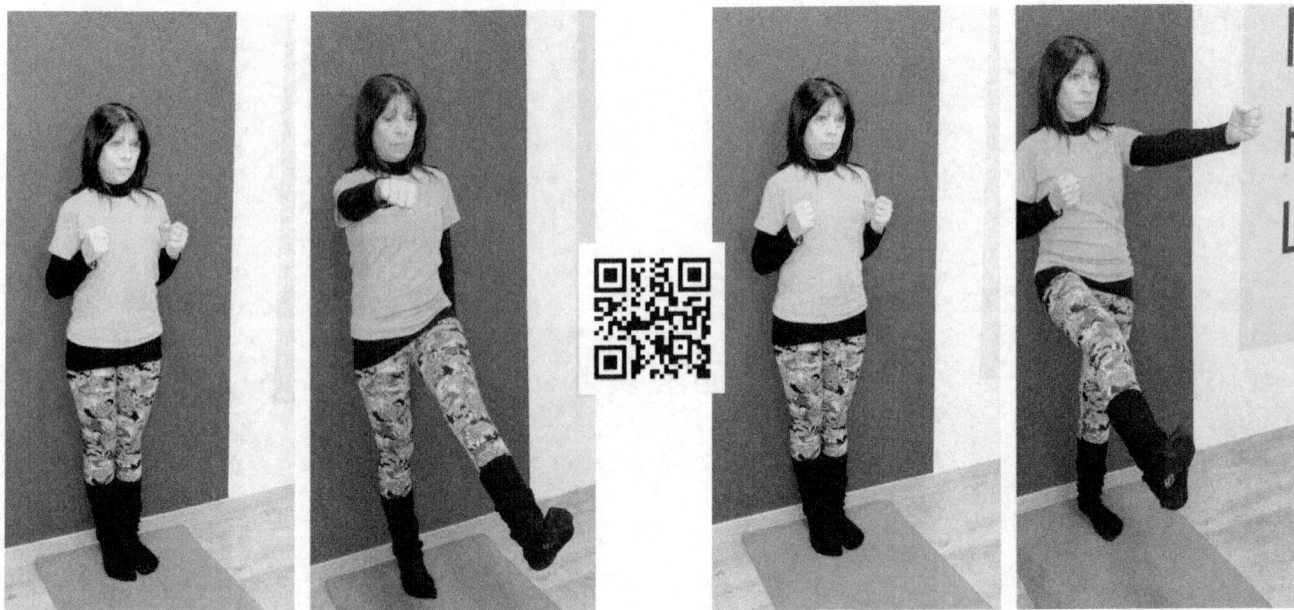

Muscles involved: A great exercise to warm up the whole body.

Level: Basic.

Execution: Stand while leaning your back and buttocks against the wall. Place your hands at chest height and keep your feet together. Strike forward with your right hand and simultaneously kick with your left leg. Repeat the movement on the other side.

Common Mistakes: Not alternating sides, holding your breath, pulling away from the wall.

Tips: Inhale at the beginning of the movement and exhale as you begin to punch forward.

KNEE RAISE WITH WALL SUPPORT (CARDIO, STRENGTH)

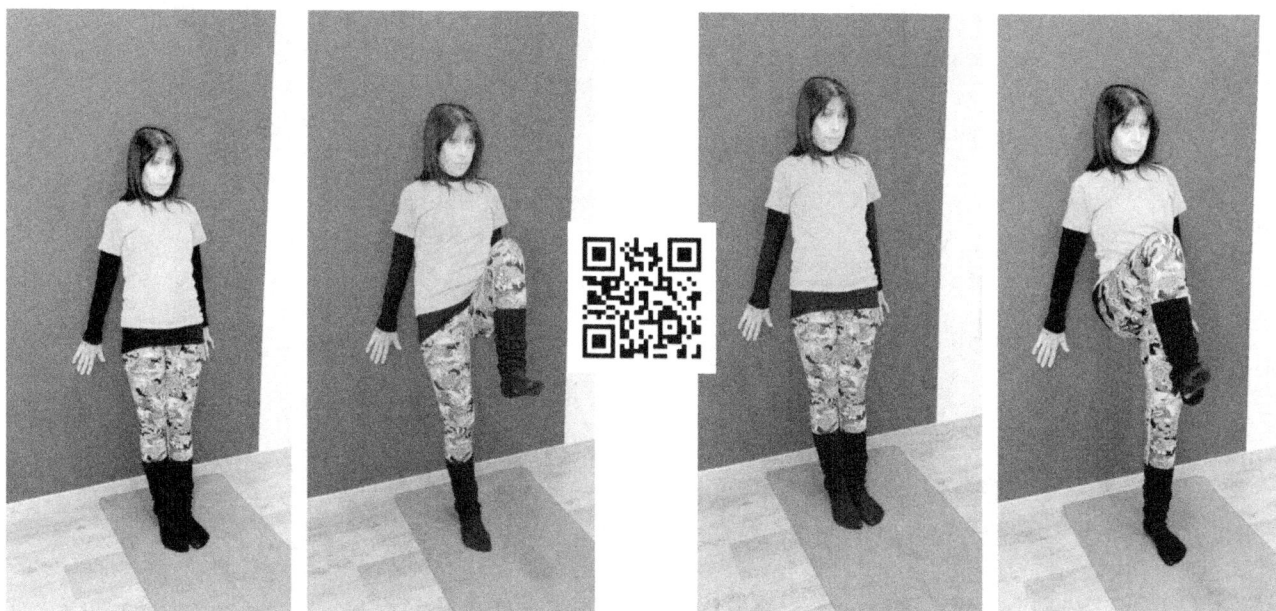

Muscles involved: Hip flexors and lower abdominals.

Level: Basic.

Execution: Lean your upper back against the wall. Place your feet forward and keep them together. Ensure your arms and hands are leaning against the wall for extra support. From there, lift your left knee to your upper limit. Return to the starting position. Perform the movement with the other knee, alternating knees.

Common Mistakes: Holding your breath, not alternating legs, not standing against the wall.

Tips: To make the exercise more challenging, try doing it with ankle weights.

PUSH BACK TO THE WALL (CARDIO, 'CORE')

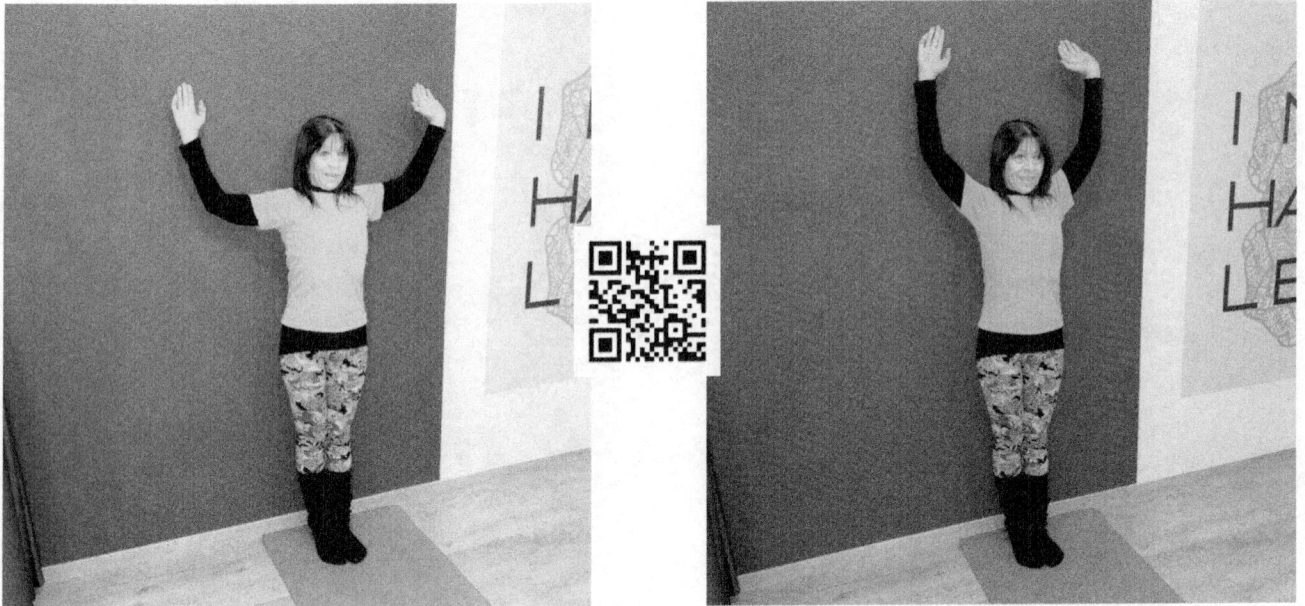

Muscles Involved: A fantastic exercise that improves posture and stimulates the shoulders and muscles of the middle back.

Level: Basic.

Execution: Stand up straight against the wall with your buttocks, head, and upper back fixed to the wall. Open your arms, keeping them resting against the wall. Bend your elbows to a 90-degree angle, palms facing forward. Slide your arms up the wall, past your shoulders, then come down and slide your elbows down along your sides. Perform multiple repetitions.

Common Mistakes: Disengaging the elbows from the wall, holding your breath, going too fast.

Tips: If you lack enough mobility, you can step away from the wall. Also, you can gently bend your knees to flatten your back even more.

MOUNTAIN CLIMBER (CARDIO, 'CORE')

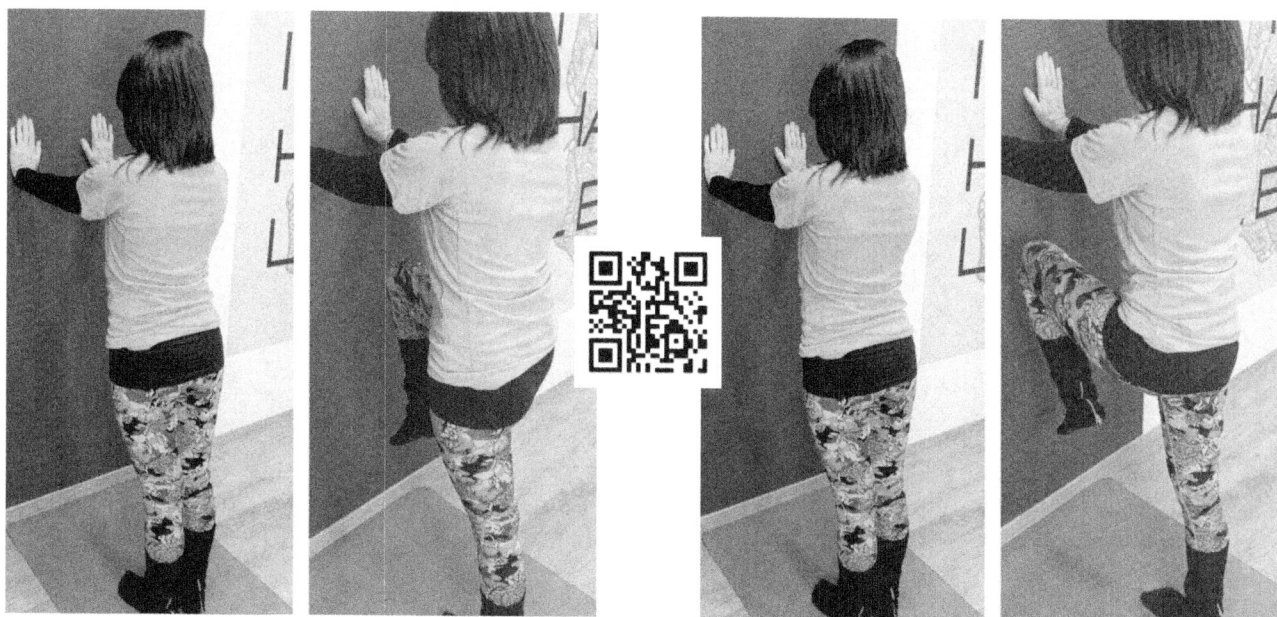

Muscles involved: An excellent exercise that works the cardiovascular system, improving overall fitness level.

Level: Basic.

Execution: Stand upright with your feet shoulder-width apart. Rest your hands on the wall for support, keeping your arms outstretched. Lift one knee, lower it, and then raise the other. Keeping your back straight, repeat the movement.

Common Mistakes: Performing the movement on one side only, holding your breath.

Tips: You can increase the intensity of this exercise by alternating legs much faster.

19. "CORE" AND STRENGTH EXERCISES

BIKE CRUNCH ('CORE,' STANDING)

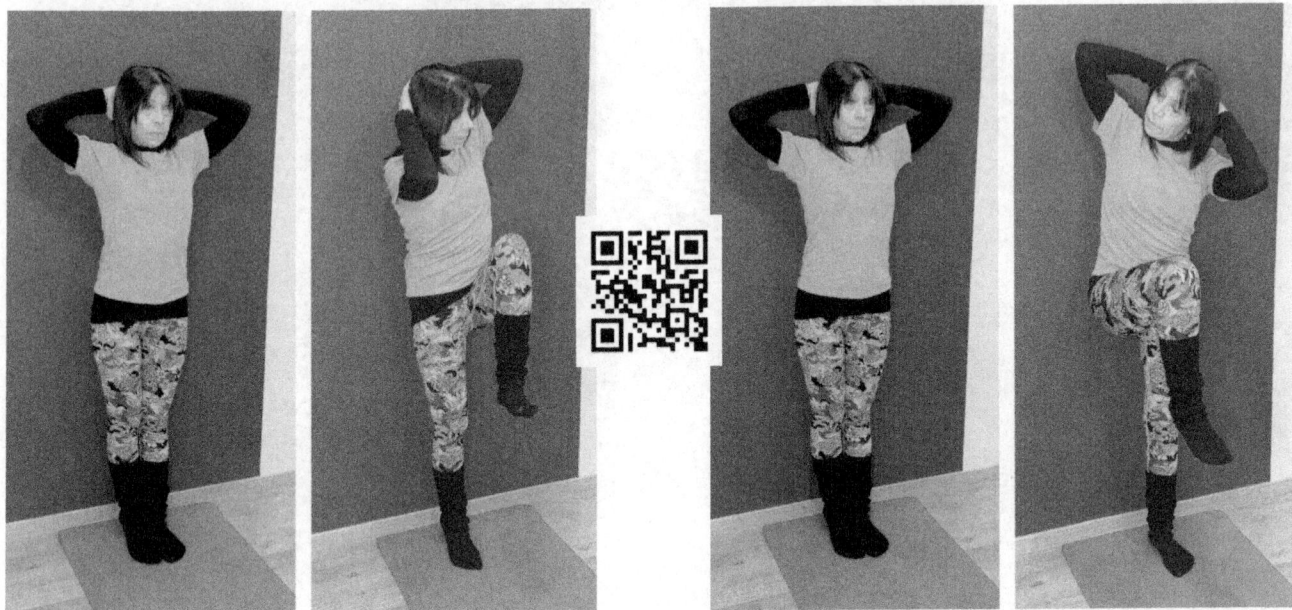

Muscles involved: Excellent exercise for working the abdominal muscles.

Level: Intermediate.

Execution: Stand while leaning your back and buttocks against the wall. Place both hands behind your head. Keep your feet together. Raise your left knee and simultaneously bring your right elbow toward your knee. Lower the knee and bring the elbow back to the starting position. Repeat the exercise with the right knee and left elbow.

Common Mistakes: Not standing in contact with the wall, holding your breath, not alternating sides.

Tips: Inhale at the beginning of the movement and exhale as you lift the leg.

SEATED CHEST ROTATION ('CORE,' FLEXIBILITY, SEATED)

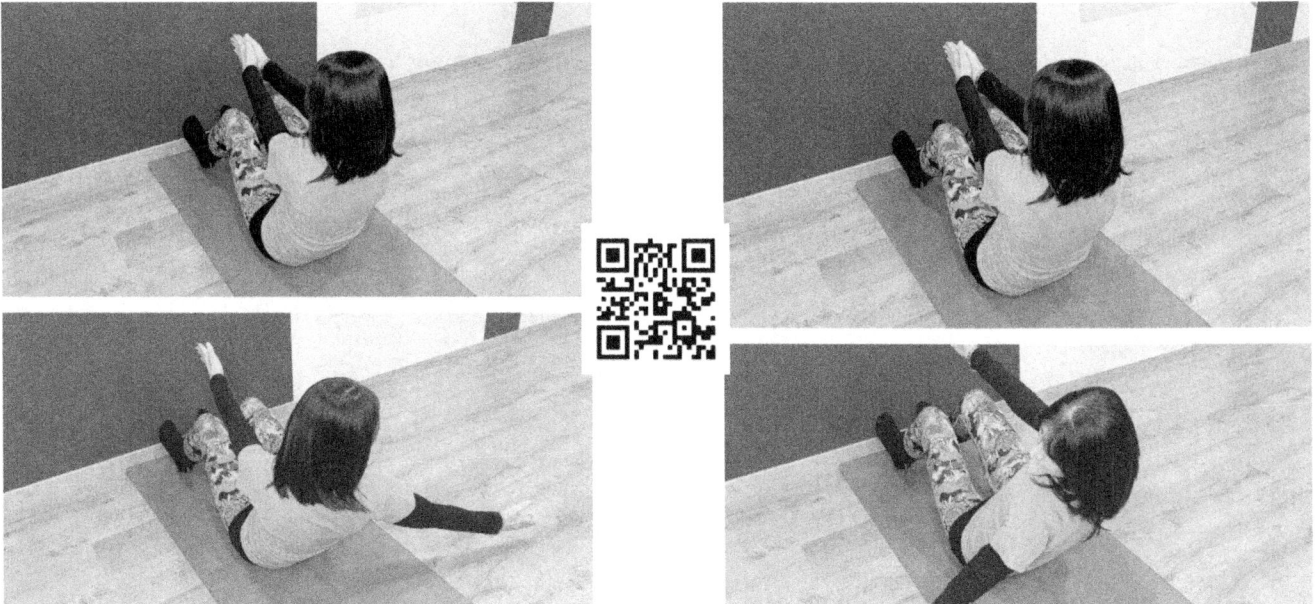

Muscles involved: Abdominals, thoracic spine mobility.

Level: Intermediate.

Execution: Sit on the floor on the mat facing the wall and place both toes on the wall. Keep your knees slightly bent and lean back a little. Bring your hands together in front of you, keeping your arms extended. From here, rotate one arm and body backward and try to touch your hand to the floor. Return to the starting position. Repeat the movement on the other side.

Common Mistakes: Rushing the movement, holding your breath.

Tips: Be sure to keep your abdominals contracted to avoid overloading the lower back.

ALTERNATING CRUNCHES WITH WALL SUPPORT ('CORE,' LYING DOWN)

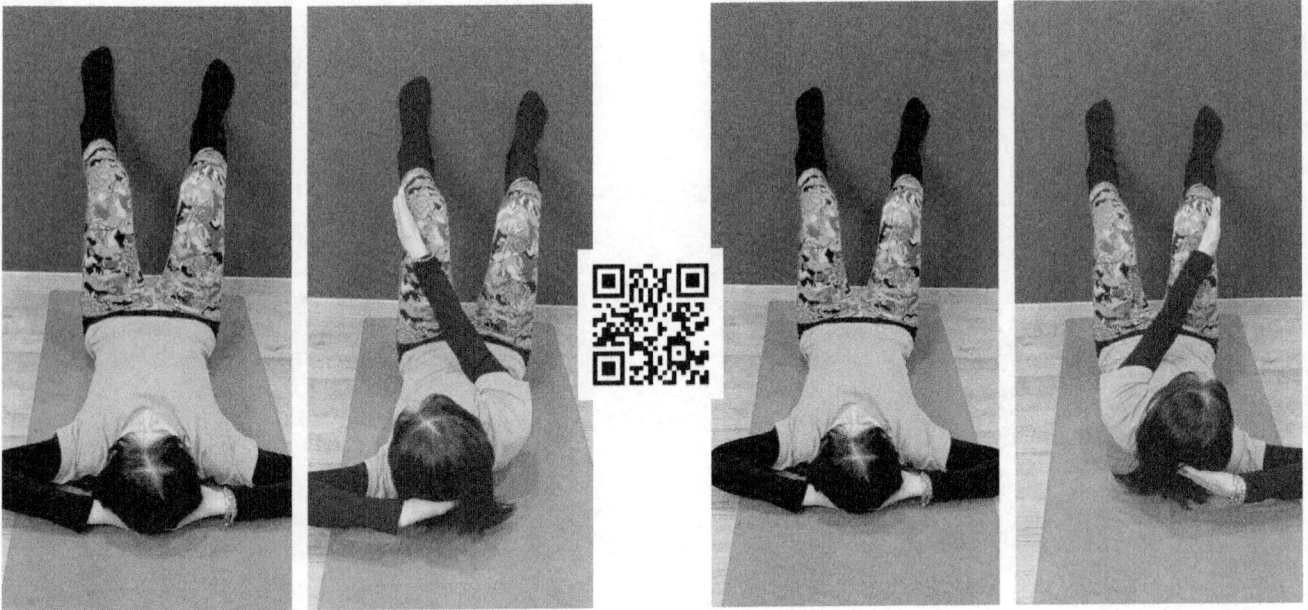

Muscles involved: Abdominals.

Level: Intermediate.

Execution: Lie on the floor on the mat with your feet on the wall. Keep your knees bent at a 90-degree angle and your feet resting on the wall, legs spread at hip width. Rest your hands behind your head. Contract your abdominals, detach your right hand from your head, extend your arm by lifting your shoulder upward, and bring your right hand to the outside of your left knee. Try to keep your left elbow steady on the floor. Lower and return to the starting position. Repeat on the other side.

Common Mistakes: Rushing the movement, not alternating sides, holding your breath.

Tips: Inhale at the beginning of the movement and exhale as you rise to perform the crunch.

WALL CRUNCHES ('CORE,' LYING DOWN)

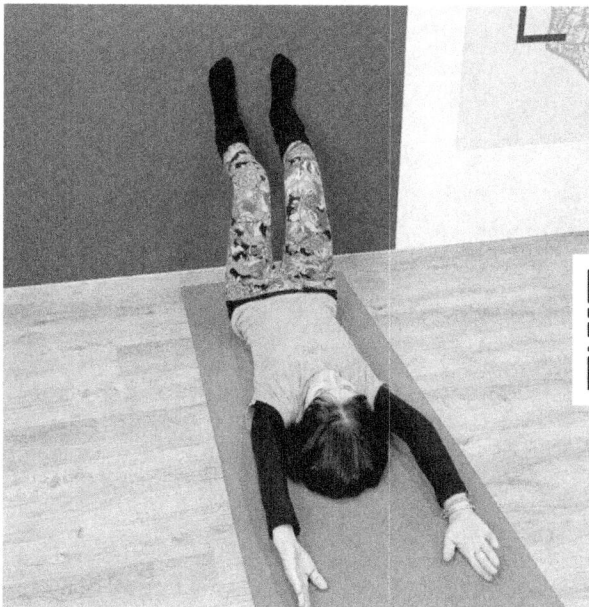

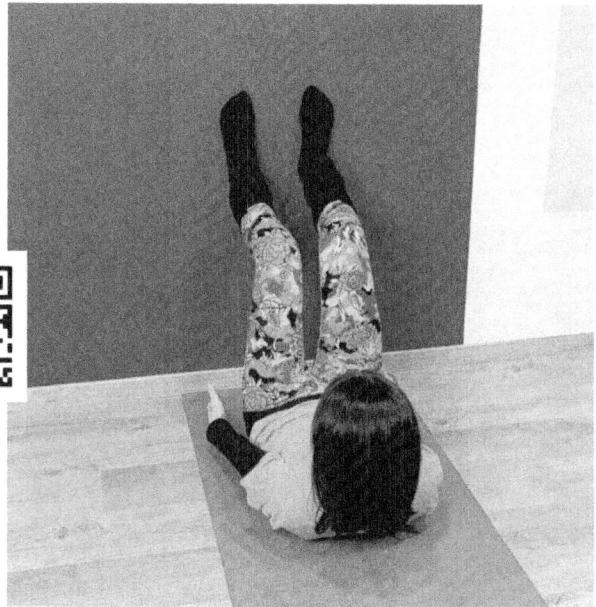

Muscles involved: A fantastic dynamic exercise to activate the abs and dynamically stretch the large back muscles.

Level: Basic.

Execution: Lie on your back on the mat. Put your knees at a 90-degree angle while resting your feet on the wall. Extend your arms back near your head. Contract your abs, bring your arms up above your head, do a crunch, lift your shoulders off the floor slightly by bending forward, and bring your arms forward until your fingers touch the floor. Slowly come back, bringing your arms up over your head, and drop to the floor until you return to the starting position.

Common Mistakes: Curling the lower back, not lifting the shoulders off the floor, giving yourself momentum.

Tips: Inhale at the beginning of the movement and exhale slowly as you begin to do the crunches. This will increase abdominal activation.

KNEE TO CHEST CRUNCH ('CORE,' LYING DOWN)

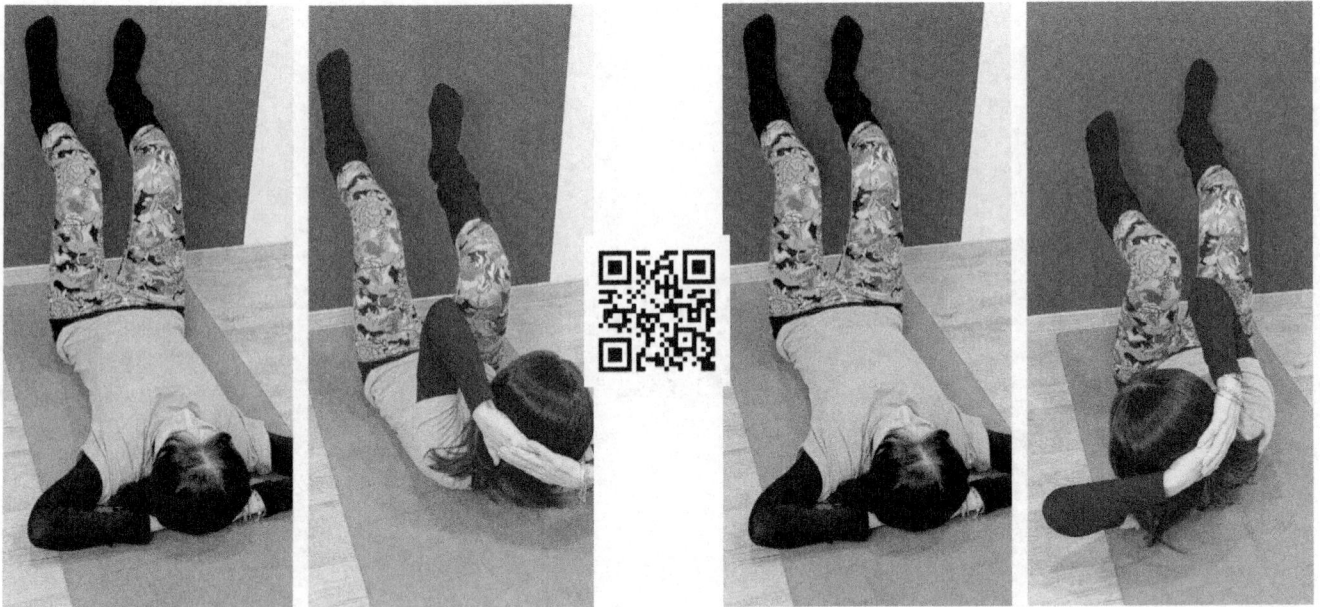

Muscles involved: An exercise that activates the hip flexors and stimulates the abdominal muscles.

Level: Basic.

Execution: Lie on your back. Put your knees at a 90-degree angle while resting your feet on the wall. Put your hands behind your head. Contract your abdominals. Simultaneously bring one knee to your chest and pull your shoulders off the floor, bringing them toward your knee. Return to the starting position. Repeat the exercise with the other knee.

Common Mistakes: Doing the movement on one side only, holding your breath, not lifting the shoulders off the floor.

Tips: Inhale at the beginning of the movement and exhale slowly as you start doing side crunches. This will increase abdominal activation.

CRUNCH WITH STRETCH ('CORE,' LYING DOWN)

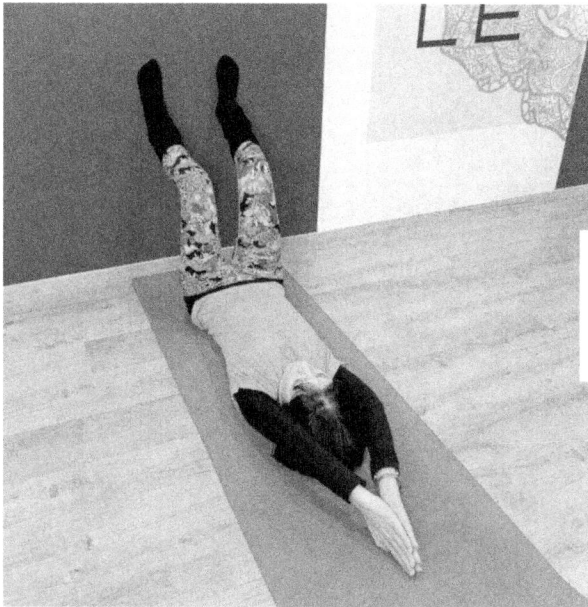

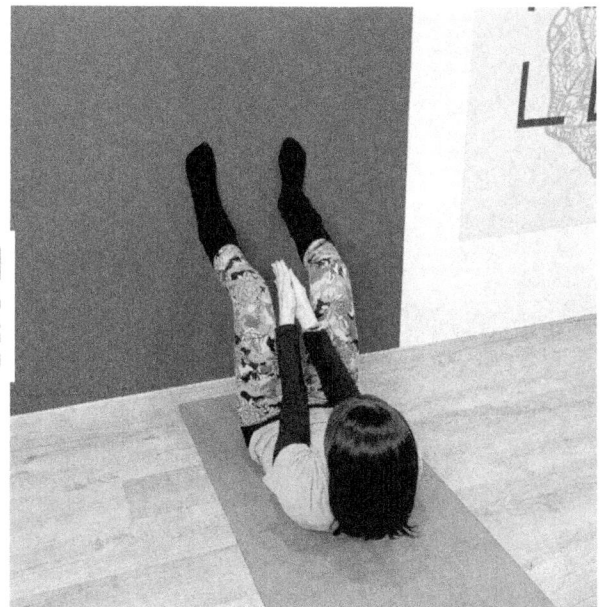

Muscles involved: An excellent exercise to activate the abs.

Level: Intermediate.

Execution: Lie on your back on the mat. Put your knees at a 90-degree angle while resting your feet on the wall. Extend your arms above your head and bring your hands together. Contract your abs, do a crunch, lift your shoulders off the floor slightly by bending forward, and bring your arms forward until your joined hands come between your knees. Slowly come back, bringing your arms up over your head, and drop to the floor until you return to the starting position.

Common Mistakes: Not lifting the shoulders off the floor, giving yourself momentum.

Tips: Inhale at the beginning of the movement and exhale slowly as you begin to do the crunches. This will increase abdominal activation.

ALTERNATE DONKEY KICK (STRENGTH, STANDING)

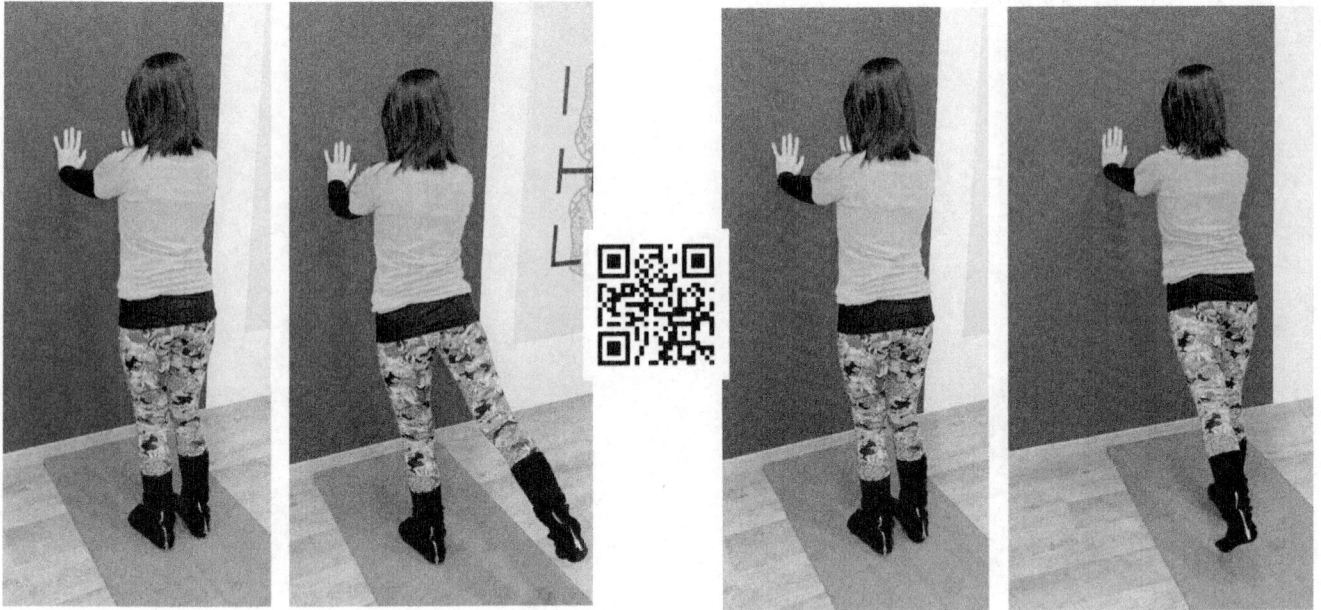

Muscles involved: Glutes and hip flexors.

Level: Basic.

Execution: Stand in front of the wall one step apart. Keep your feet together and bend your knees slightly. Place both hands on the wall. Extend one of your legs backward, then lower it and bring it back to the starting position. Perform the exercise with the other leg.

Common Mistakes: Arching the spine, not alternating sides, rushing the movement.

Tips: Maintain a regular breathing rhythm.

WALL SQUAT (STRENGTH, STANDING)

Muscles involved: Quadriceps and glutes.

Level: Basic.

Execution: Stand with your hands resting on the wall. Make sure you spread your legs slightly. Squat down as if you were sitting, forming a 90-degree angle between your back and thighs. Then return to a standing position.

Common Mistakes: Holding your breath, rushing the movement, not going down to 90 degrees.

Tips: Inhale before you start to lower, exhale when you start to rise. Contract your abdominals throughout the movement.

PRESSURE ARMS TO THE WALL PALMS FORWARD (STRENGTH, STANDING)

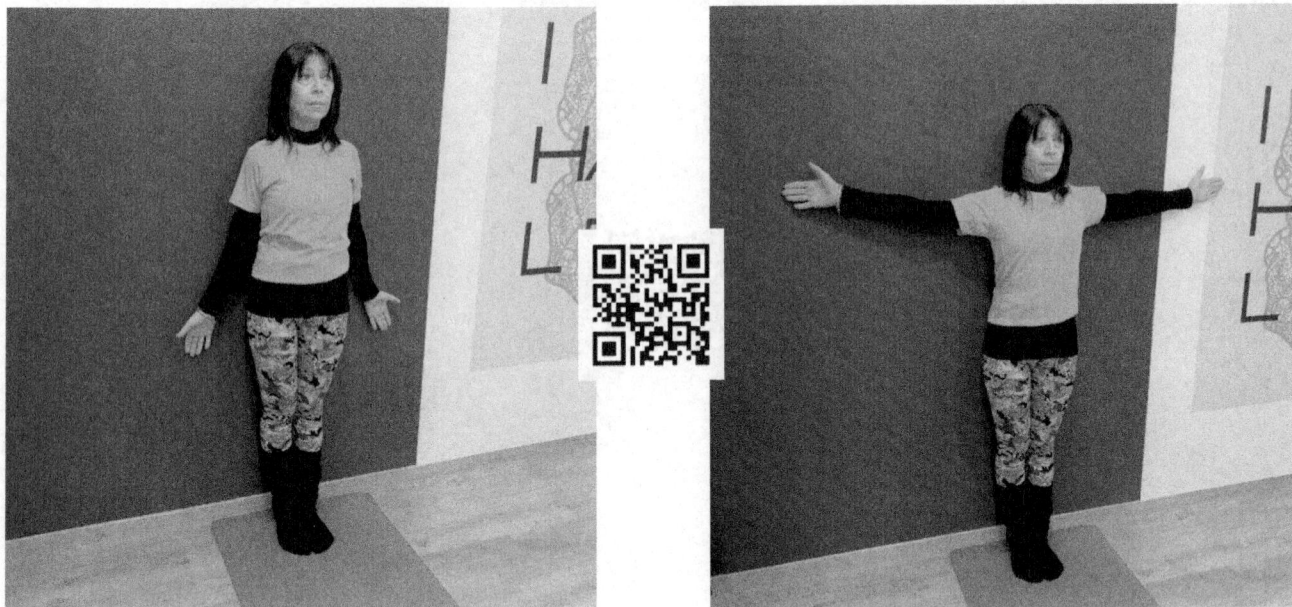

Muscles involved: Muscles of the middle back.

Level: Basic.

Execution: Stand upright with your back against the wall. Ensure your head, buttocks, and upper back are well supported against the wall. Keep your feet together. Keep your arms close to your sides. Lift your arms sideways along the wall to shoulder height. From this position, apply pressure toward the wall with the backs of your hands. Stay in this position and maintain the pressure.

Common Mistakes: Bending the arms, holding your breath, not maintaining the static position.

Tips: Inhale at the beginning of the movement and exhale during the pressure to the wall.

PRESSURE ARMS TO THE WALL PALMS TO THE WALL (STRENGTH, STANDING)

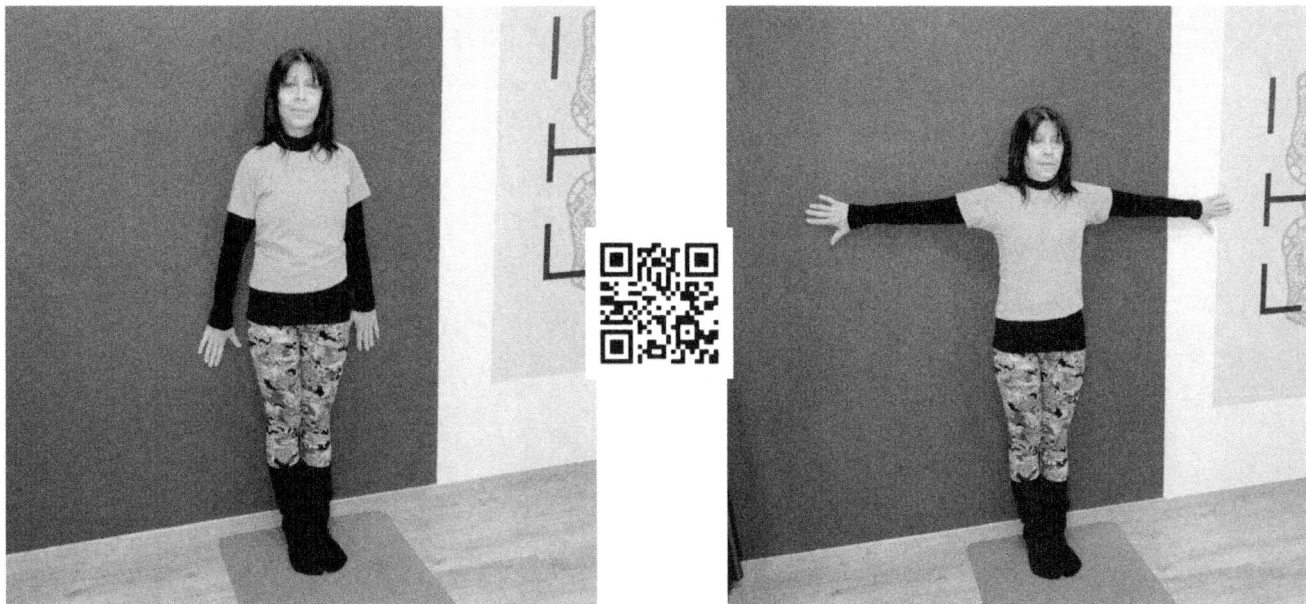

Muscles involved: Muscles of the middle back, deltoids, and triceps.

Level: Basic.

Execution: Stand upright with your back against the wall. Ensure your head, buttocks, and upper back are well supported against the wall. Keep your feet together. Keep your arms close to your sides. Lift your arms sideways along the wall to shoulder height. From this position, apply pressure toward the wall with your palms. Stay in this position and maintain the pressure.

Common Mistakes: Bending the arms, holding your breath, not maintaining the static position.

Tips: Inhale at the beginning of the movement and exhale during the pressure to the wall.

PLANK POSE WITH WALL SUPPORT (STRENGTH, STANDING)

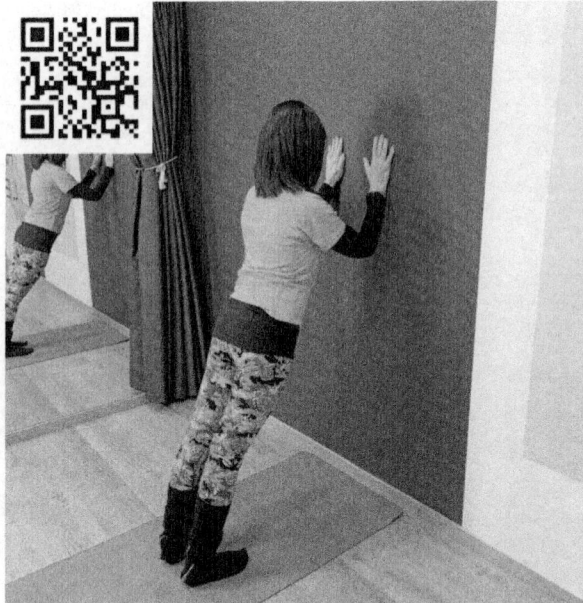

Muscles involved: Stimulates arm, shoulder, and abdominal muscles.

Level: Intermediate.

Execution: Stand facing the wall and place your hands on the wall at shoulder height. Let your elbows relax near your hips and drop toward the floor. Contracting your abdomen, step back by putting more weight on your hands. Do not let your hips fall toward the wall. Hold the position and inhale and exhale deeply 2-3 times.

Common Mistakes: Letting the pelvis fall forward, holding the breath.

Tips: Inhale deeply 2-3 times as long as you hold the position.

SQUAT WITH STANCE CHANGE (STRENGTH, STANDING)

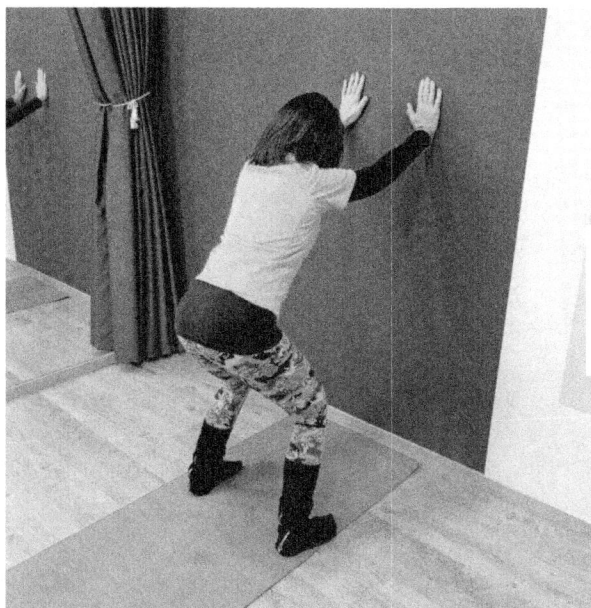

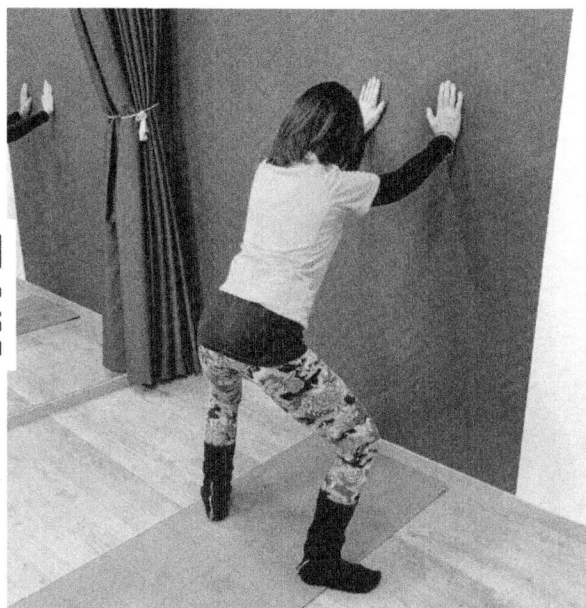

Muscles involved: Quadriceps and glutes.

Level: Intermediate.

Execution: Stand one step away from the wall. Place your hands on the wall. Spread your feet slightly apart. Squat down and as you stand up rotate your toes outward while keeping your heels on the ground. Squat down again. When you stand up, perform the toes rotation in reverse and return with your feet to the previous position. Continue the exercise by alternating the position of the feet with each lift of the body.

Common Mistakes: Holding your breath, rushing the movement, not going down to 90 degrees.

Tips: Inhale before you start to lower, exhale when you start to rise. Contract your abs throughout the movement.

WALL SIT (STRENGTH, STANDING)

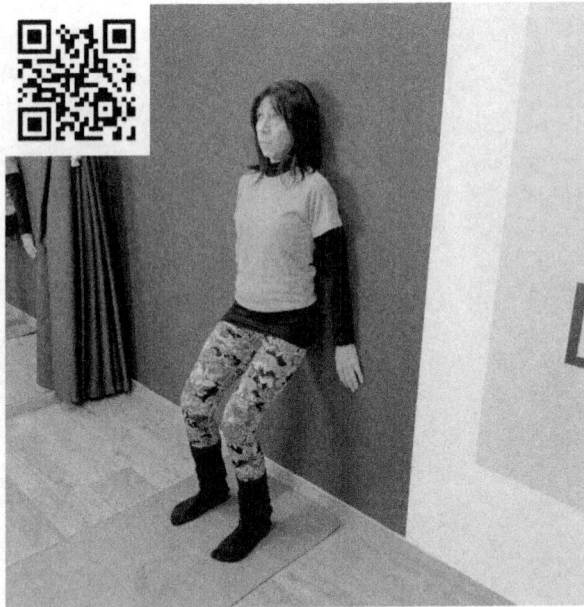

Muscles involved: This exercise strengthens the quadriceps muscles in addition to benefiting the ankles and quadriceps tendons.

Level: Intermediate.

Execution: Lean your upper back against the wall. Come

 down by sliding your back against the wall until your knees are bent at a 90-degree angle. Hold the position and breathe deeply 2-3 times.

Common Mistakes: Holding your breath, rushing the movement, disengaging the upper back from the wall.

Tips: Maintain a regular breathing pattern.

WALL PUSH UPS (STRENGTH, STANDING)

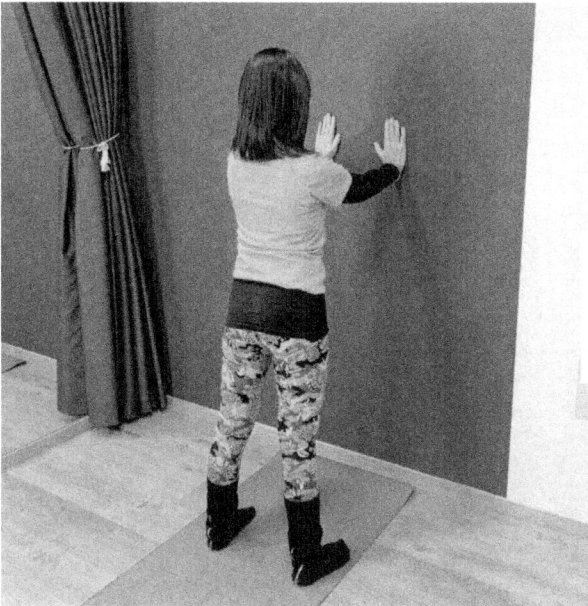

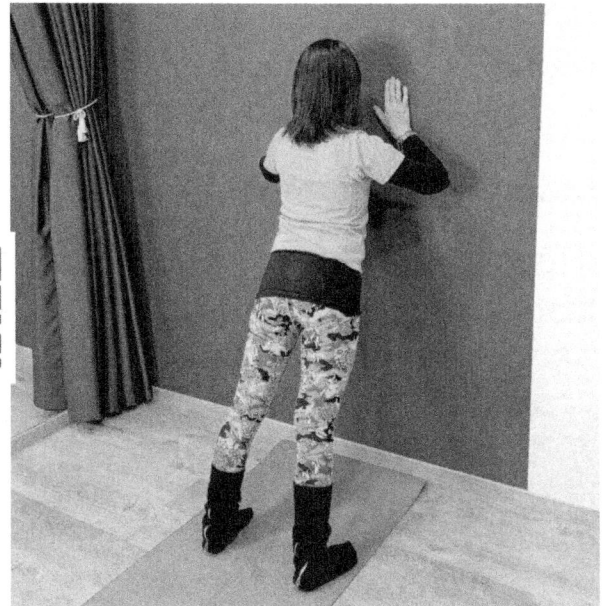

Muscles involved: Pectorals and triceps, hamstring strengthening.

Level: Intermediate.

Execution: Stand upright and bring your feet together. Rest your hands on the wall at chest height, with arms extended. From this position, bend your elbows and try to bring your chest closer to the wall. Reach your upper limit, then push with your arms and return to the starting position.

Common Mistakes: Holding your breath.

Tips: Inhale at the beginning of the movement and exhale as you begin to push back.

SEMI LUNGES WITH WALL SUPPORT (STRENGTH, STANDING)

Muscles involved: Strengthens leg muscles and improves balance.

Level: Intermediate.

RIGHT Execution: Stand in front of the wall. Place both hands on the wall. Bring your right foot forward so your toes touch the wall. Bring your left foot back one step. Step downward with your body, bending both legs forward slightly to 45 degrees. Step up and return to the starting position.

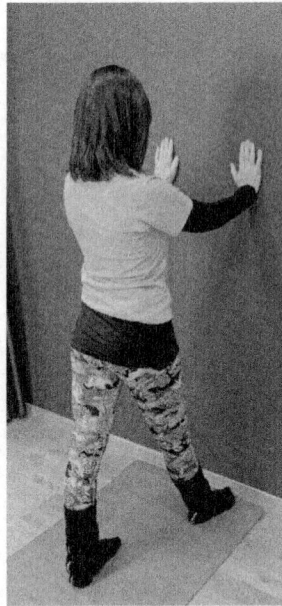

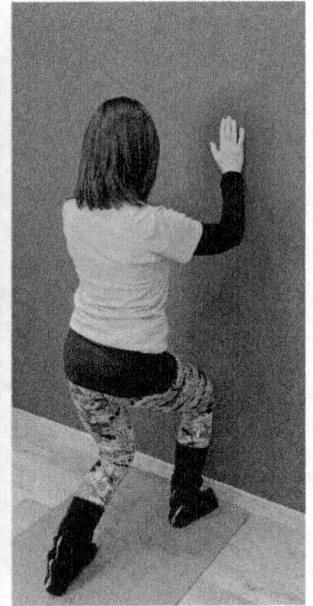

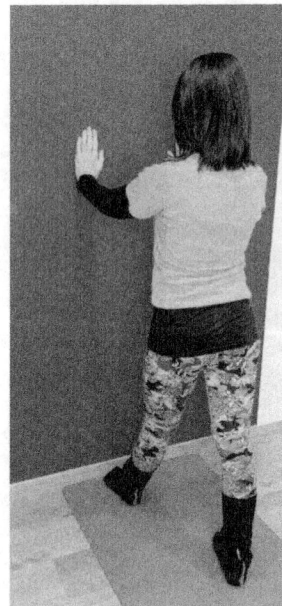

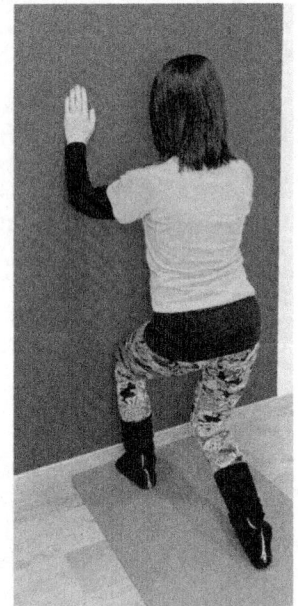

LEFT Execution: Stand in front of the wall. Place both hands on the wall. Bring your left foot forward so your toes touch the wall. Bring your right foot back one step. Step downward with your body, bending both legs forward slightly to 45 degrees. Step up and return to the starting position.

Common Mistakes: Descending too low, holding your breath, rushing the movement.

Tips: Inhale at the beginning of the movement and exhale when you come down.

ELEVATED BRIDGE (STRENGTH, LYING DOWN)

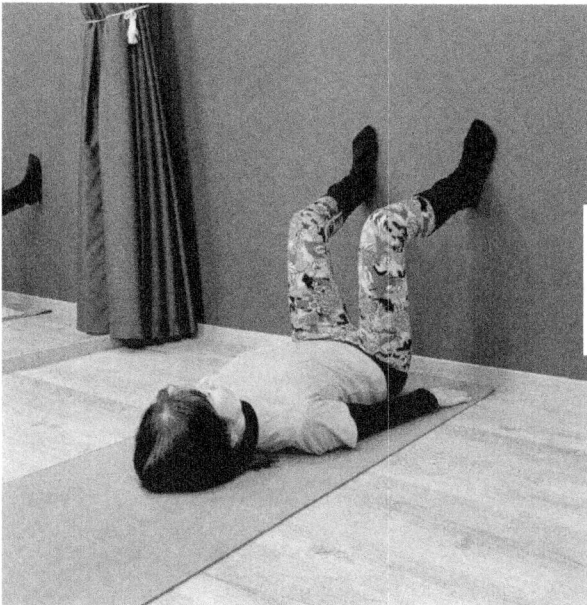

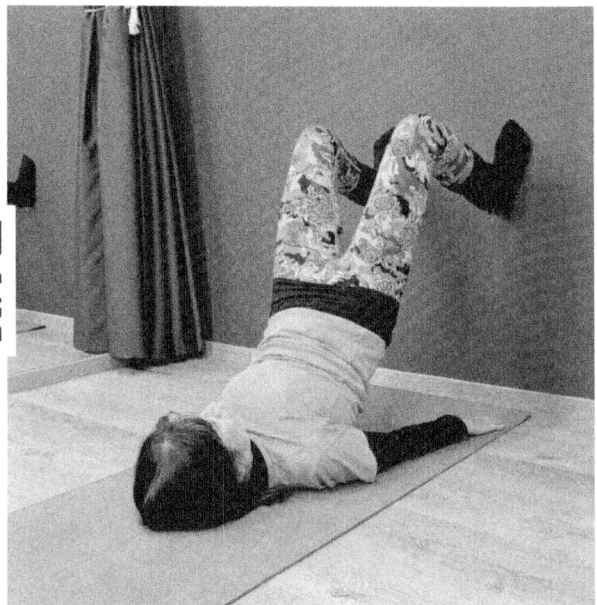

Muscles involved: Femoral and glutes.

Level: Intermediate.

Execution: Lie on the floor on a mat and rest your feet on the wall. Your legs should be slightly apart. Keep your knees bent at a 90-degree angle. Your arms and hands are extended on the floor along your sides, palms facing the floor. Lift your hips and buttocks to your full limit. Slowly return to the starting position and repeat the exercise. Your hands on the floor provide support.

Common Mistakes: Holding your breath, giving yourself momentum.

Tips: Inhale at the beginning of the movement and exhale as you come back.

ANGEL TO THE WALL (STRENGTH, MOBILITY, STANDING)

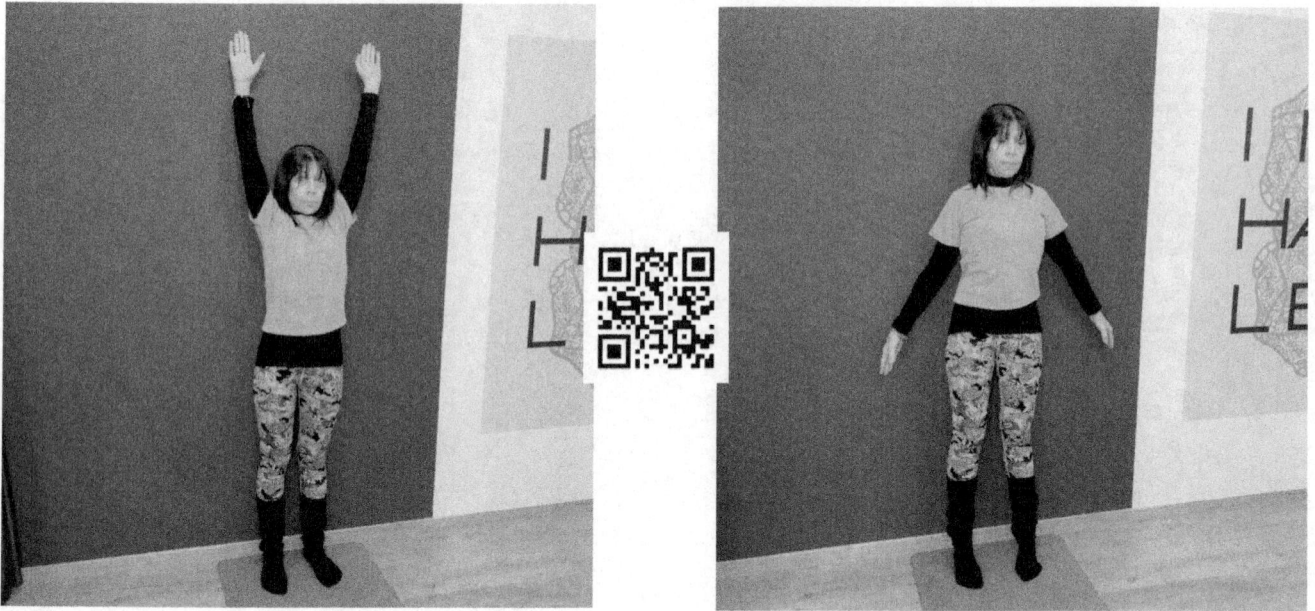

Muscles involved: Shoulder mobility and strengthening upper back muscles.

Level: Basic.

Execution: Stand up straight with feet together, back well against the wall. Extend your arms above your head, ensuring your upper back, forearms, wrists, and buttocks touch the wall. Lift your heels and, simultaneously, slide your elbows down near your hips along the wall. Your hands and wrists should slide, touching the wall. Now lower your heels and, at the same time, raise your arms, sliding them in the opposite direction from before, so they are positioned above your head.

Common Mistakes: Rushing the movement, losing contact with the wall, holding your breath.

Tips: Inhale at the beginning of the movement and exhale slowly as you lift your heels upward.

TOUCH SHOULDER-TO-WALL (STRENGTH, MOBILITY, STANDING)

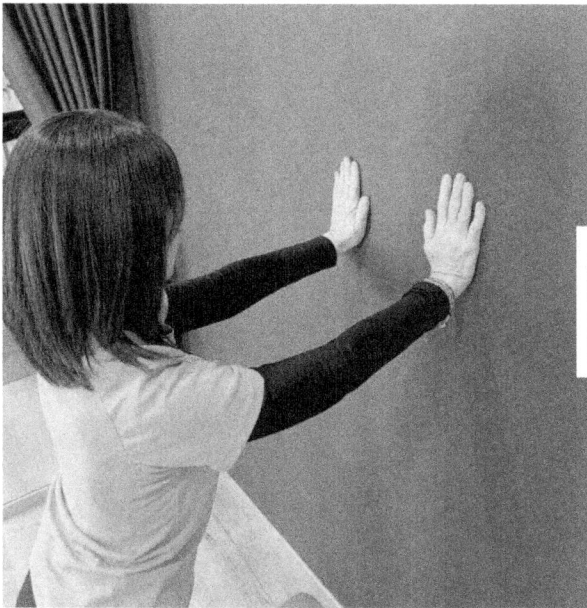

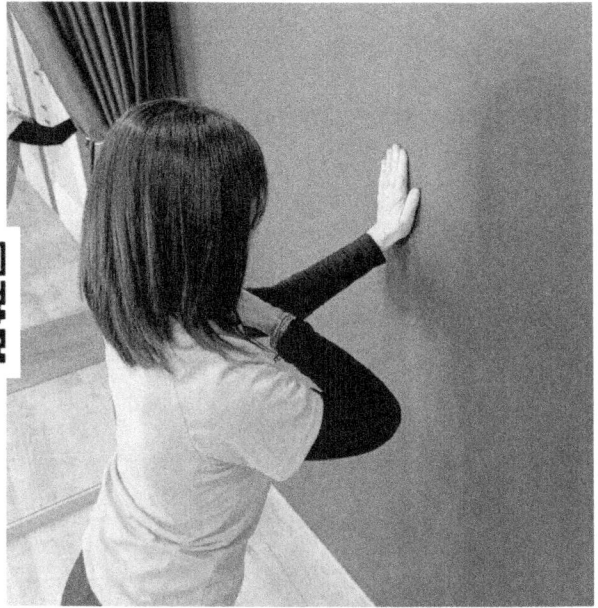

Muscles involved: Improves shoulder stability while minimally straining the rest of the body.

Level: Basic.

Execution: Stand a couple of steps away from the wall, facing it. Rest your hands on the wall at chin height, with arms slightly flexed. Keep your feet together and your abdomen contracted. Touch your right shoulder with your left hand. Return to the starting position. Perform a small forward bend with the body. Repeat on the other side.

Common Mistakes: Not alternating sides, holding your breath, arching the spine, not keeping the core contracted.

Tips: Keep a regular breathing rhythm.

DONKEY KICKS AND WALL CURL (STRENGTH, MOBILITY, STANDING)

Muscles involved: Glutes, femoral muscles.

Level: Basic.

RIGHT Execution: Stand a little away from the wall. Rest your hands on the wall. Keep your feet together. Extend your right leg backward and upward without bending the knee. Lower the right leg to the starting position, then bend the right knee, trying to bring the heel as close as possible to the gluteus. Return to the starting position and start over.

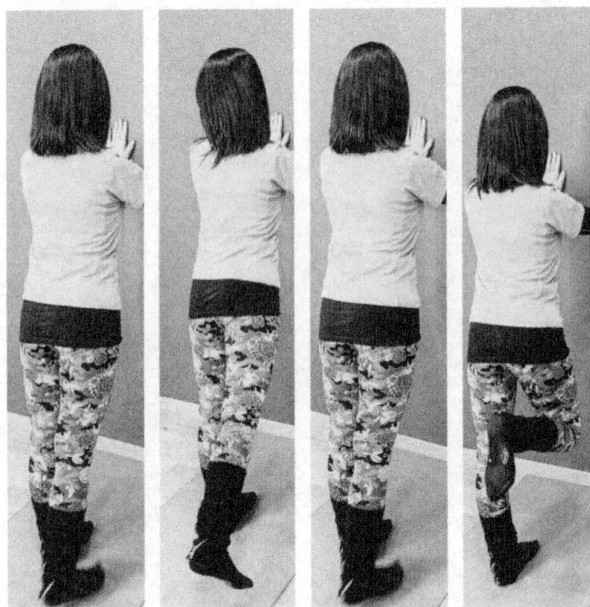

LEFT Execution: Stand a little away from the wall. Rest your hands on the wall. Keep your feet together. Extend your left leg backward and upward without bending the knee. Lower the left leg to the starting position, then bend the left knee, trying to bring the heel as close as possible to the buttock. Return to the starting position and start over.

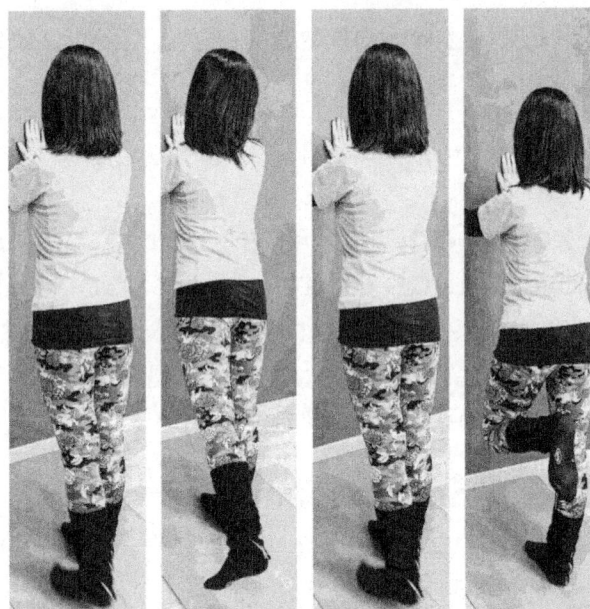

Common Mistakes: Arching the spine, rushing the movement, holding the breath, bending the knee during the backward momentum of the leg.

Tips: Inhale at the beginning of the movement and exhale while continuing.

LEG CIRCLE (STRENGTH, MOBILITY, STANDING)

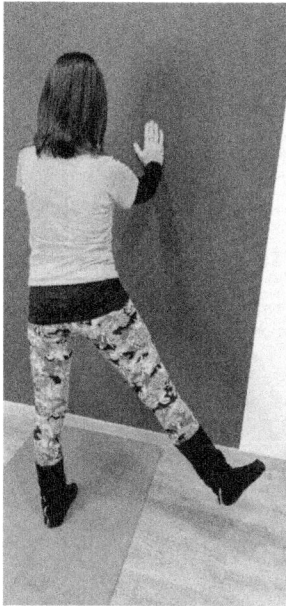

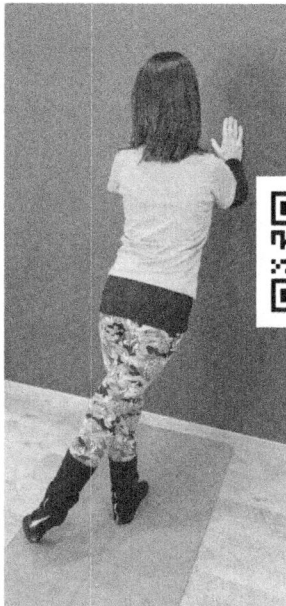

Muscles involved: Hip mobility and gluteal toning.

Level: Basic.

RIGHT Execution: Stand in front of the wall one step away. Keep your feet together and bend your knees slightly. Place both hands on the wall. Extend your right leg to the side, then lift it up and bring it behind your left leg, to the side. Return to the starting position and repeat the exercise.

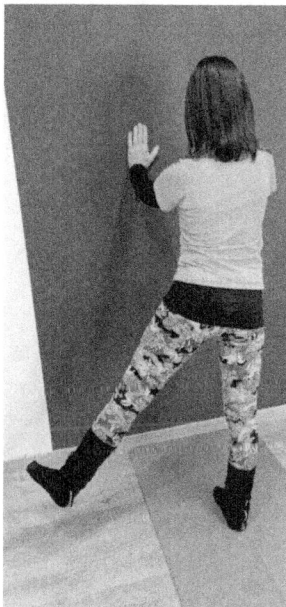

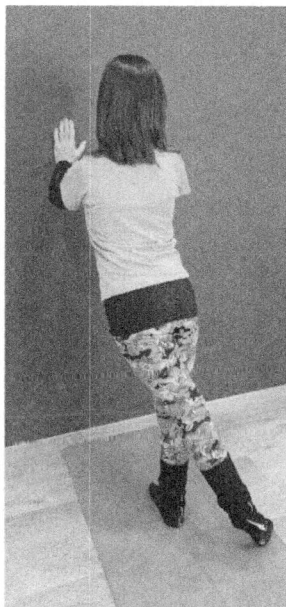

LEFT Execution: Stand in front of the wall one step away. Keep your feet together and bend your knees slightly. Place both hands on the wall. Extend your left leg to the side, then lift it up and bring it behind your right leg, to the side. Return to the starting position and repeat the exercise.

Common Mistakes: Holding your breath, rushing the movement, arching the spine.

Tips: Maintain a regular breathing rhythm.

20. BALANCE EXERCISES

LEG LATERAL THRUST (BALANCE, STRENGTH, STANDING)

Muscles involved: Glutes.

Level: Basic.

RIGHT Execution: Stand sideways to the wall with the left side of your body. Place your left hand on the wall and your right hand on your side. Keep your feet together. Without bending your body, lift your right leg sideways with thrust then return to the starting position.

LEFT Execution: Stand sideways to the wall with the right side of your body. Place your right hand on the wall and your left hand on your side. Keep your feet together. Without bending your body, lift your left leg sideways with thrust then return to the starting position.

Common Mistakes: Bending your knees, bending your body as you lift your leg, holding your breath.

Tips: Maintain a regular breathing rhythm.

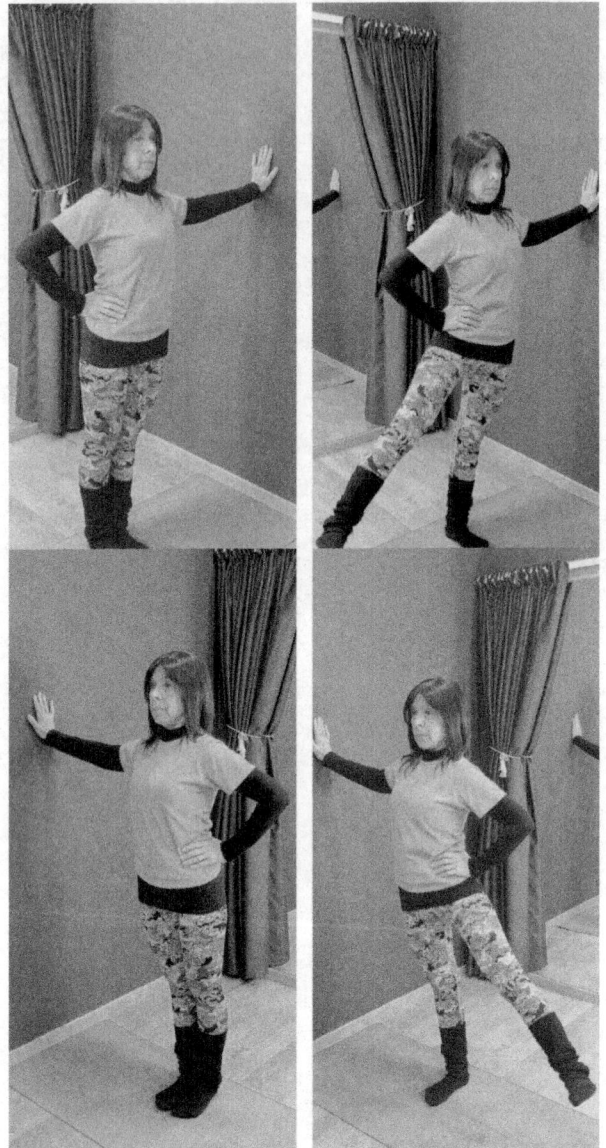

STANDING SIDE CRUNCHES (BALANCE, 'CORE,' STANDING)

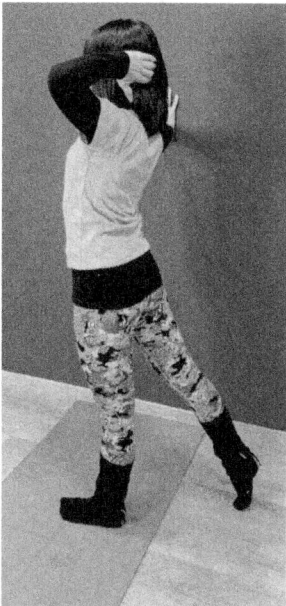

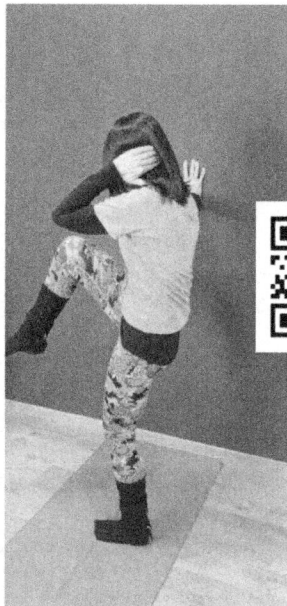

Muscles involved: Improves core strength, hip flexors, and stability.

Level: Intermediate.

RIGHT Execution: Stand sideways to the wall, place your right hand on the wall, and your left hand behind your head. Move your right leg back, resting your toe on the ground. From there, raise your right knee toward your chest and bring your left elbow toward your right knee. Return to the starting position.

LEFT Execution: Stand to the side of the wall, place your left hand on the wall, and your right hand behind your head. Move your left leg back, resting your toe on the ground. From there, raise your left knee toward your chest and bring your right elbow toward your left knee. Return to the starting position.

Common Mistakes: Rushing the movement, holding your breath, arching the back backward.

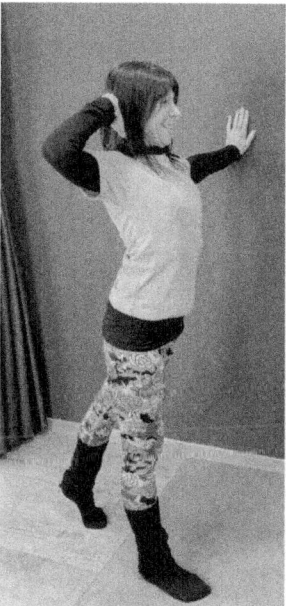

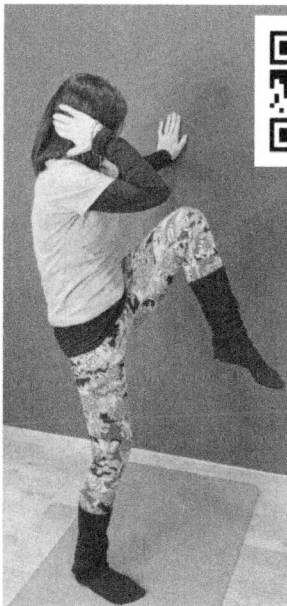

Tips: Inhale when both feet are on the ground, exhale as you bring your knee toward your chest.

BIRD DOG POSE WITH WALL SUPPORT (BALANCE, STRENGTH, 'CORE,' QUADRUPED)

Muscles involved: Improves core strength, hip flexors, and stability. A fantastic exercise that activates the posterior chain and core while also challenging stability.

Level: Basic.

RIGHT Execution: Use a mat and stand on all fours to the side of the wall, with the wall to your left. Contract your abdominals. Place your knees well under your hips and your hands under your shoulders. Extend your left arm and right leg simultaneously. Do not rush; perform the exercise slowly. Gaze toward the floor, not forward, to keep the spine straight. Try to keep your balance; your right hip should not fall.

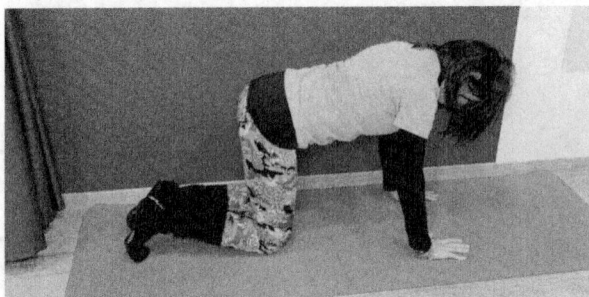

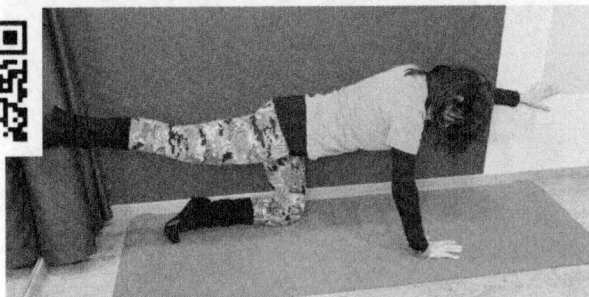

LEFT Execution: Use a mat and stand on all fours to the side of the wall, with the wall to your right. Contract your abdominals. Place your knees well under your hips and your hands under your shoulders. Extend your right arm and left leg simultaneously. Perform the exercise slowly. Gaze toward the floor, not forward, to keep the spine straight. Try to keep your balance; your left hip should not fall.

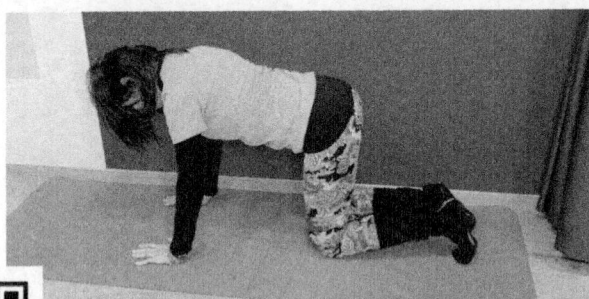

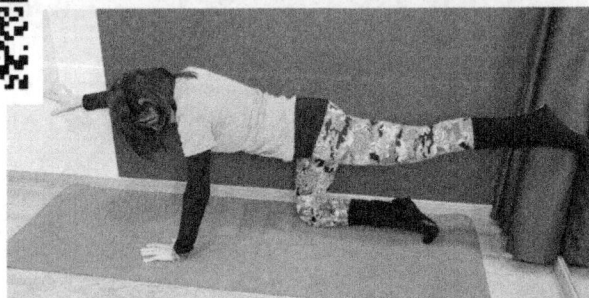

Common Mistakes: Bending the lower back, rushing the movement.

Tips: Perform this movement slowly. Contract your abs before starting.

PIGEON POSITION WITH WALL SUPPORT (BALANCE, STRENGTH, STANDING)

Muscles involved: Strengthens joints, leg muscles, and buttocks.

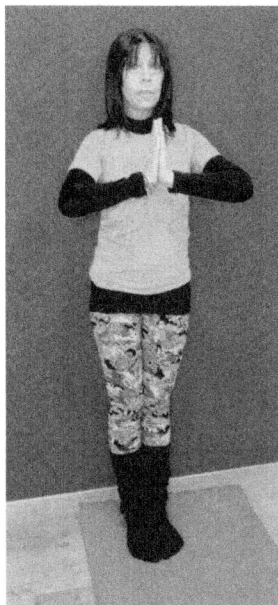

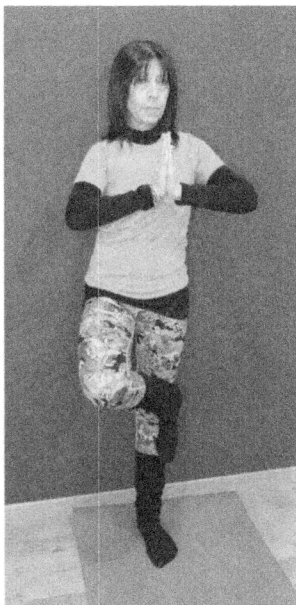

Level: Intermediate.

Execution: Position yourself with your back against the wall. Take a couple of breaths and rotate your shoulders back and forth to create flexibility. Stand erect with relaxed shoulders and chin parallel to the ground. Keep your legs firmly planted, close together, and straight. Bring your palms together at heart height, feeling the force in the calves, ankles, and thigh muscles. Inhale and keep your left foot firmly on the mat. Lift your right leg and place your right foot on your left knee. Breathe calmly and concentrate on maintaining balance. Stay as long as possible, then release. Repeat with the right leg on the ground and the left foot on the right knee, staying as long as you can.

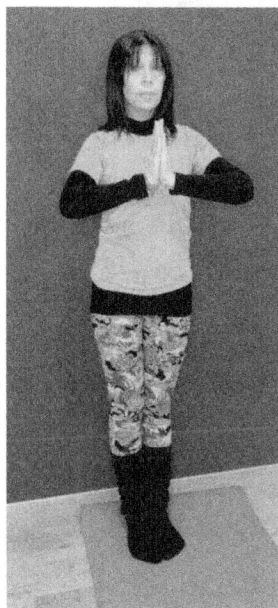

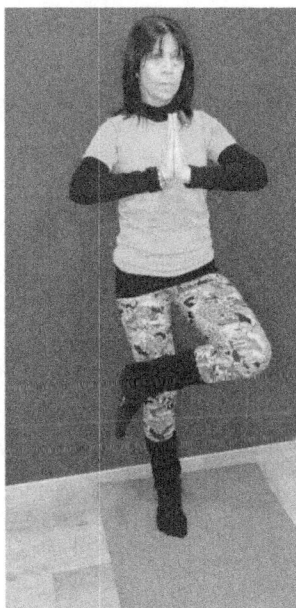

Common Mistakes: Holding your breath.

Tips: Fixate on a focal point to maintain balance. Advanced students can close their eyes if they feel secure.

21. FLEXIBILITY, STRETCHING AND DEFATIGUE EXERCISES

SEATED SIDE BENDS (STRETCHING, SEATED)

Muscles involved: Stretching lower back muscles and side abdominals.

Level: Basic.

Execution: Sit on the floor on the mat with your back properly resting against the wall. Spread your legs apart. Bend your body to the left side while extending your right arm above your head, bringing it toward the toes of your left foot. Hold the position for a few seconds. Return to the starting position and then perform the exercise on the other side.

Common Mistakes: Holding your breath, rushing the movement, bending the legs and arms.

Tips: Inhale at the beginning of the movement, exhale when you start bending to the side.

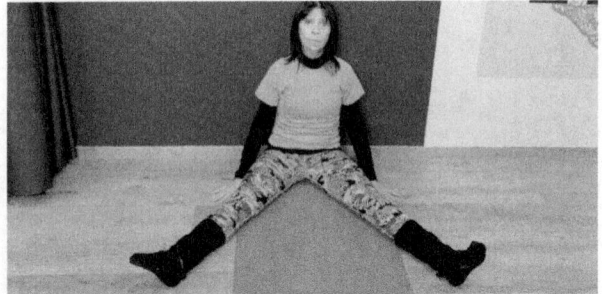

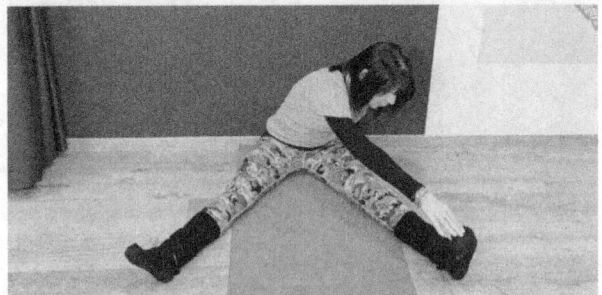

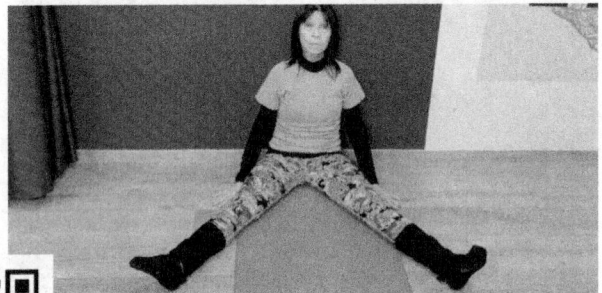

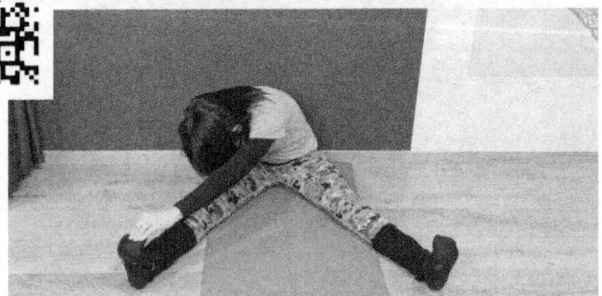

STANDING KNEE LIFT (STRETCHING, FLEXIBILITY, STANDING)

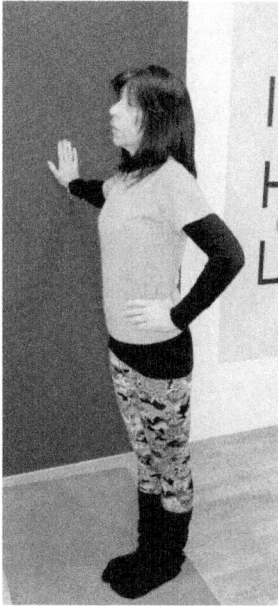

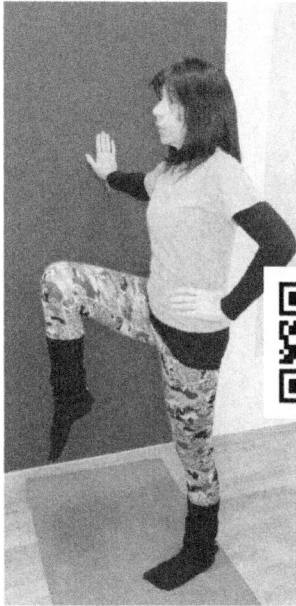

Muscles involved: Hip flexors and stability improvement.

Level: Basic.

RIGHT Execution: Stand sideways to the wall with your right hand on the wall and your left hand on your hip. Lift your right knee, lower it, and bring it back to the starting position. Repeat the movement.

LEFT Execution: Stand sideways to the wall with your left hand on the wall and your right hand on your hip. Lift your left knee, lower it, and bring it back to the starting position. Repeat the movement.

Common Mistakes: Rushing the movement, bending the lower back, holding your breath.

Tips: To make this exercise more challenging, add light ankle weights.

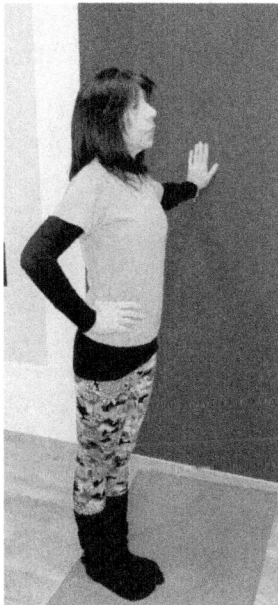

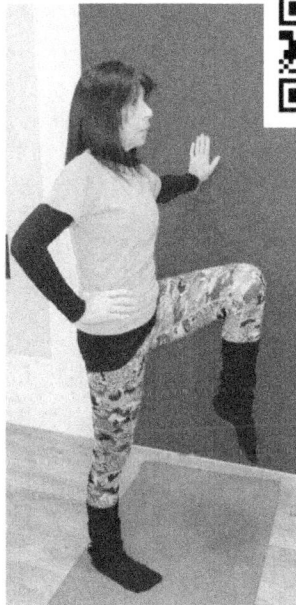

FACE-DOWN DOG POSE (STRETCHING, FLEXIBILITY, STANDING)

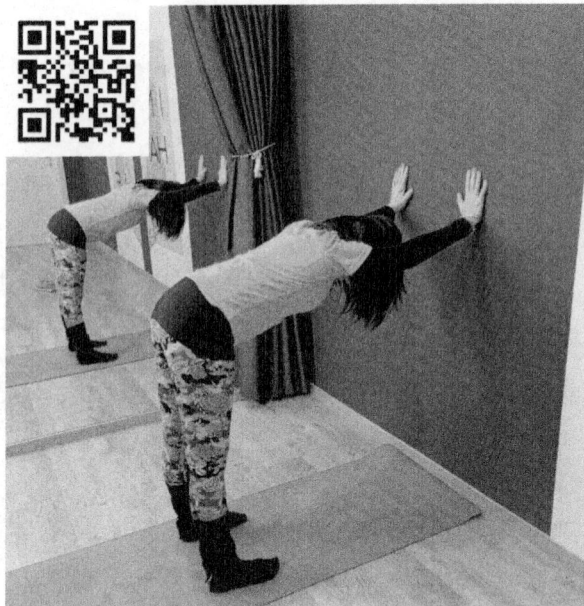

Muscles involved: This excellent exercise stretches the hamstrings and decompresses the lower back.

Level: Basic.

Execution: Keep your feet slightly wider than shoulder-width apart. Push your hips back and rest your hands on the wall. Slowly lower your chest and head into your arms, keeping your torso parallel to the floor. Maintain the stretch.

Common Mistakes: Bending your arms or legs, holding your breath, bending the lower back.

Tips: Inhale at the beginning of the movement and exhale slowly once parallel to the floor. Continue to inhale and exhale deeply while holding the position.

COBRA POSE (STRETCHING, FLEXIBILITY, STANDING)

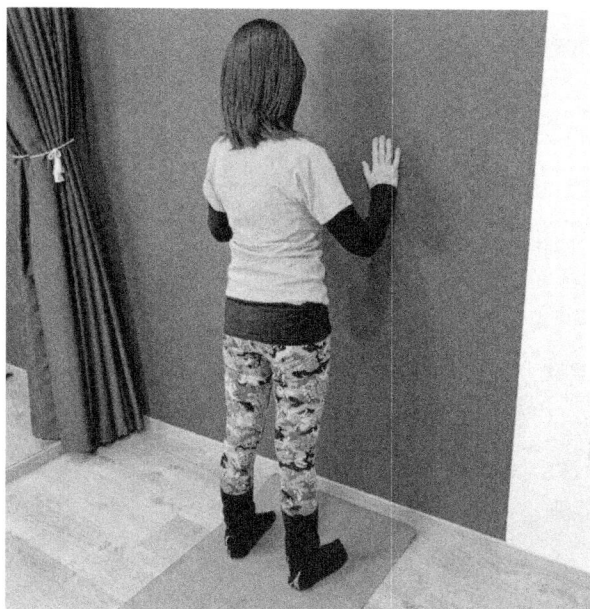

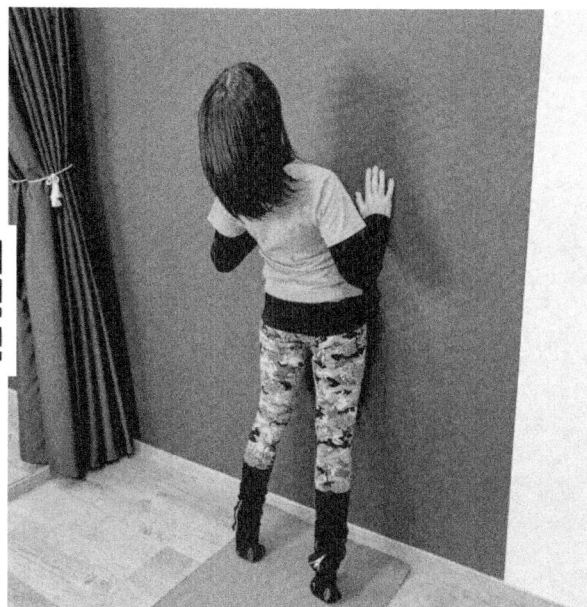

Muscles involved: Arm, shoulder, and back muscles.

Level: Intermediate.

Execution: Stand a few inches from the wall. Place your hands on the wall at shoulder height for support, elbows along your sides. Inhale and press your feet into the floor. Now exhale, lifting your chest up and bending backward. Slowly look up and then back as you press your pelvis against the wall. Inhale and rise onto your tiptoes while pressing your pelvis against the wall and bringing your shoulders back as far as you can. Exhale and lower your feet to the floor, slowly returning to the starting position.

Common Mistakes: Holding your breath, disengaging your pelvis from the wall, lifting elbows away from your sides.

Tips: You can skip rising onto your tiptoes when first performing this exercise.

ACTIVE FROG STRETCH (STRETCHING, FLEXIBILITY, ON ALL FOURS)

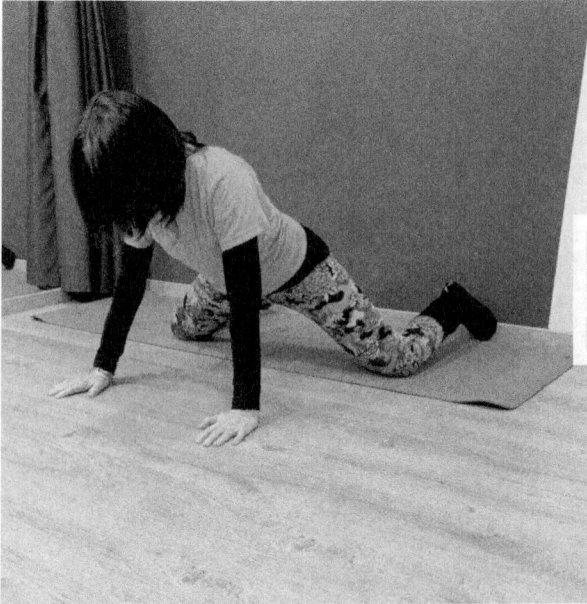

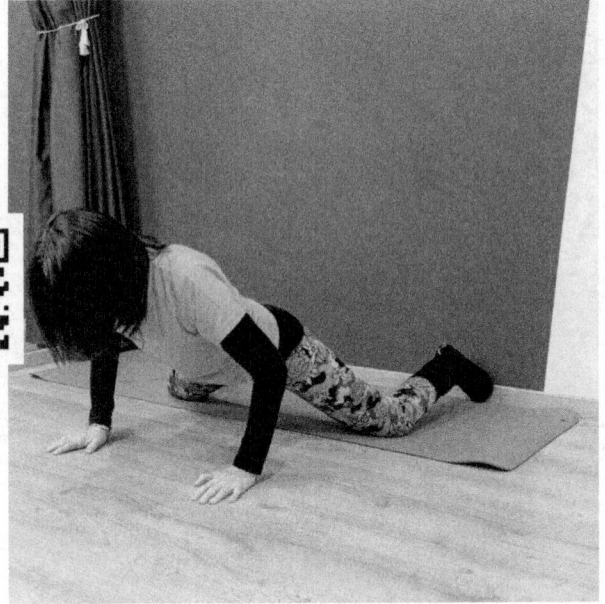

Muscles involved: This exercise is a dynamic stretch for the adductor muscles. It can also improve hip mobility. It's really useful as a warm-up before squats.

Level: Basic.

Execution: Position yourself on the floor on the mat on all fours, leaning on your hands. Open your knees as wide as possible. Rest the tips of your feet against the wall. Move your body forward and back. Keep your lower back straight.

Common Mistakes: Curving the lower back, not keeping the knees wide enough.

Tips: Maintain a consistent breathing pattern while performing this movement.

SEATED TOUCH TOES (STRETCHING, FLEXIBILITY, SEATED)

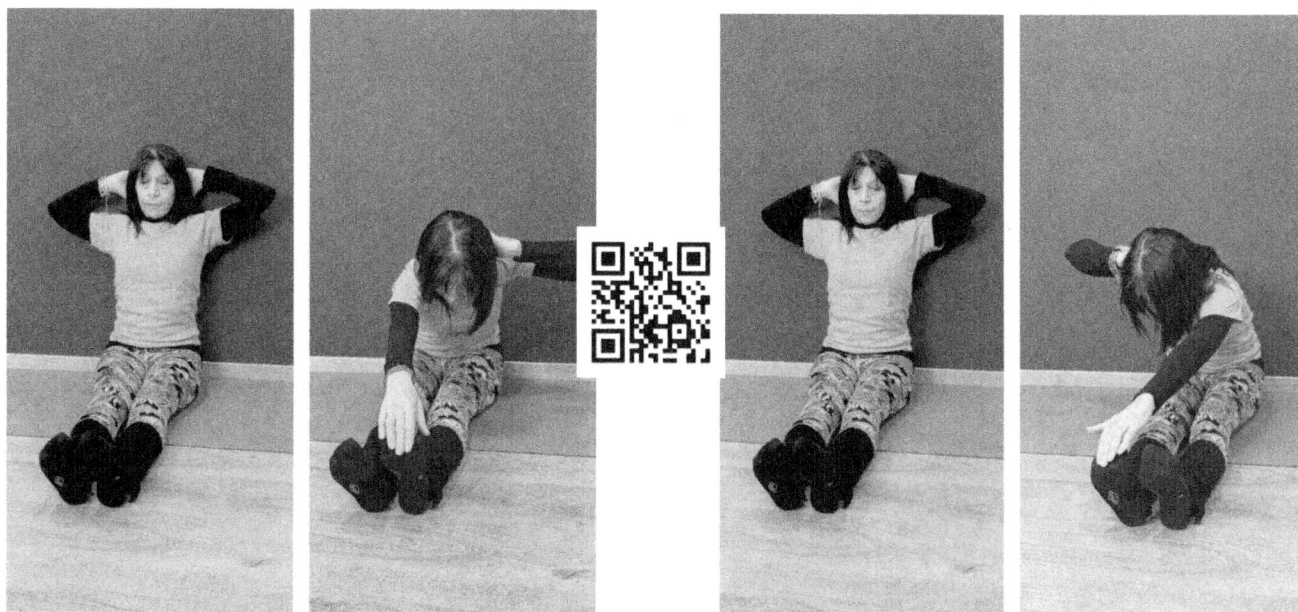

Muscles involved: A great exercise that will stretch the spinal erector muscles. Besides stretching the back, it will also stretch the hamstrings and calves.

Level: Basic.

Execution: Sit upright and lean your back against the wall. Place your hands behind your head. Keep your legs extended forward. From there, extend your left hand towards the tip of your right foot. Keep your right arm bent behind your head. Return to the starting position and do the same on the other side, right hand towards left foot. Repeat the exercise, alternating sides. Even if you don't reach your foot, that's okay; reach your limit.

Common Mistakes: Performing the movement on one side only, bending the knees, holding your breath.

Tips: Inhale at the beginning of the movement and exhale slowly as you reach towards your toes.

STRETCHING LEGS APART TO THE WALL (STRETCHING, FLEXIBILITY, LAY DOWN)

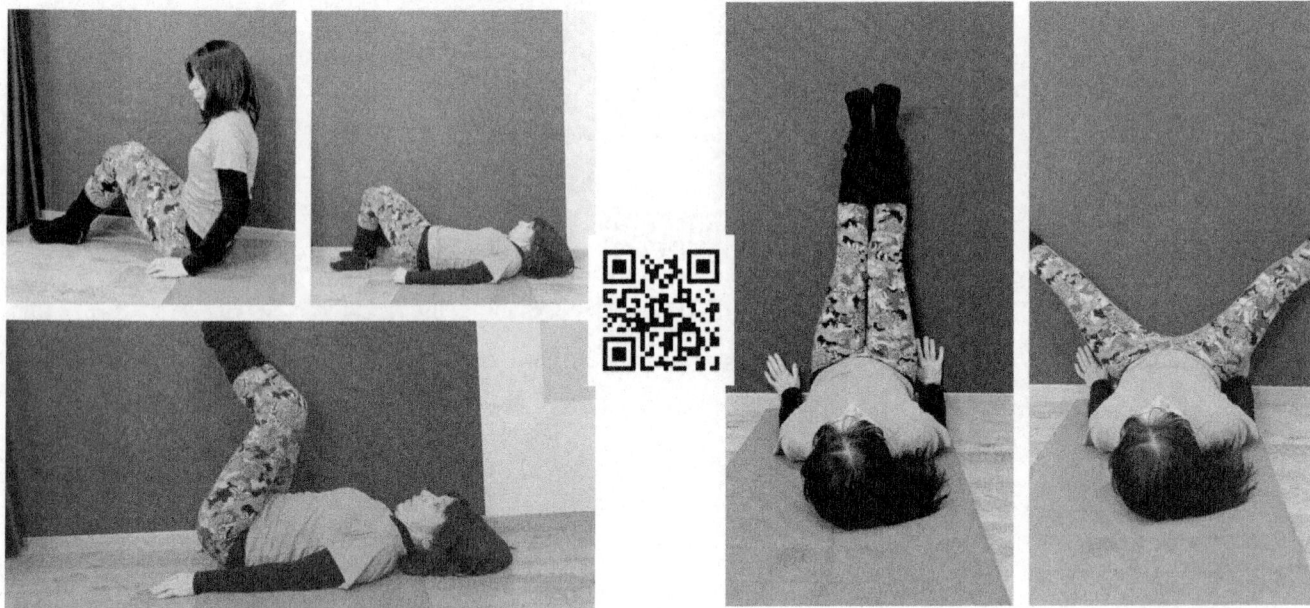

Muscles involved: This is a fantastic exercise that will stretch the adductor muscles.

Level: Basic.

Execution: To begin, sit on the floor on the mat with a shoulder near the wall and your thighs parallel to the wall. Roll back while swinging your legs onto the wall until you are lying on your back. Extend your legs up the wall, even with your buttocks against the wall. Keep your hands near your hips. Spread your legs as wide as you can and hold the static position.

Common Mistakes: Holding your breath, curving the lower back.

Tips: Maintain a consistent breathing pattern while performing this movement.

CROSSING-LEGS LYING DOWN (STRETCHING, FLEXIBILITY)

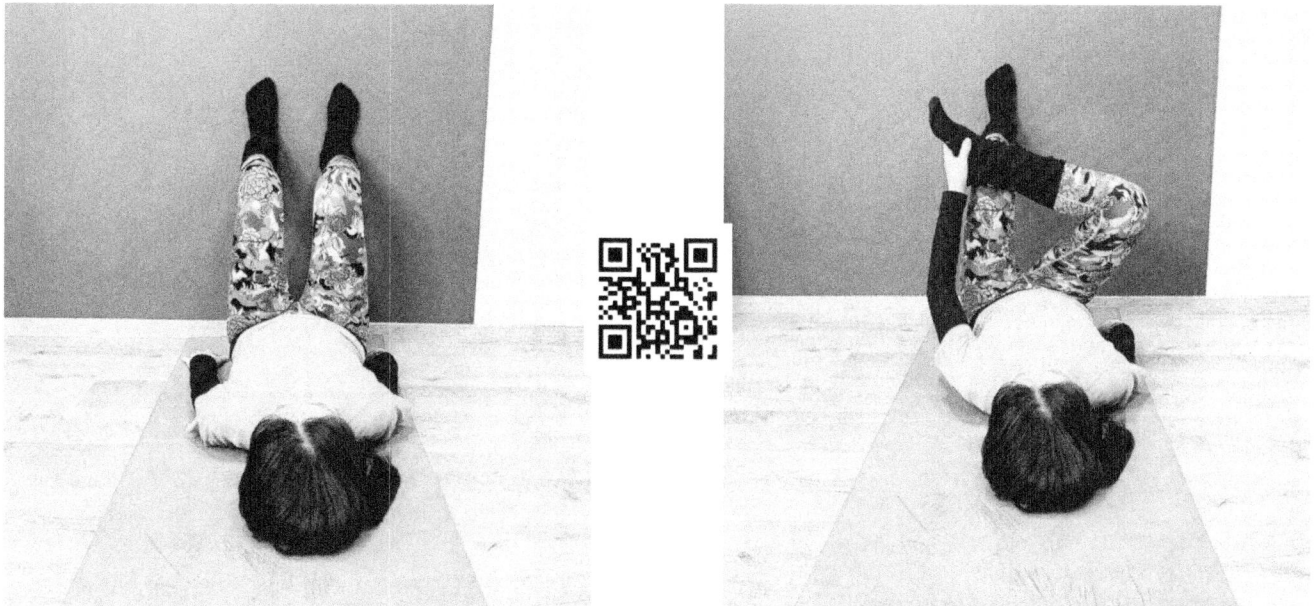

Muscles involved: An excellent exercise that works on the external rotation of the hip. Great for keeping hip joints healthy.

Level: Basic.

Execution: Lie on your back on the mat. Place your knees at a 90-degree angle, resting your feet on the wall. Bring your right knee to your chest, keeping your head and back firmly on the floor. Grab your right ankle with your left hand. Rotate your right hip and place your right foot on your left knee. Hold the position. Then change legs.

Common Mistakes: Letting the pelvis move, holding your breath, curving the lower back.

Tips: Maintain a consistent breathing pattern while performing this movement.

RAISED LEGS POSE WITH HEELS ON WALL (STRETCHING, FLEXIBILITY, LYING DOWN)

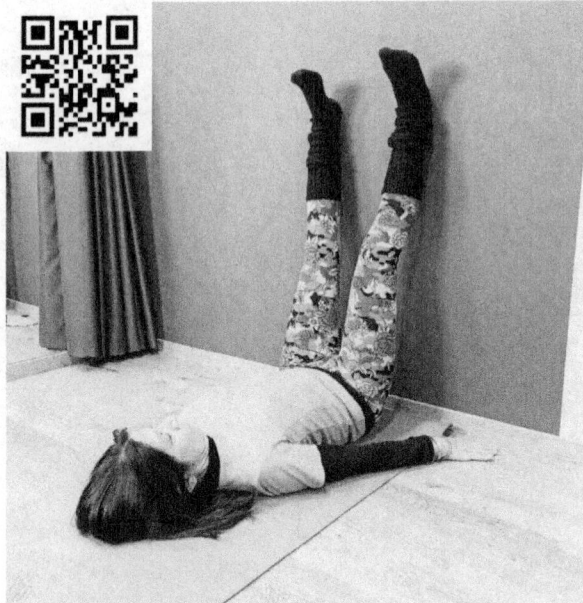

Muscles involved: Lower back, hamstrings.

Level: Basic.

Execution: To start, sit on the floor on the mat with a shoulder near the wall and your thighs parallel to the wall. Roll back, swinging your legs onto the wall. Once in position, make sure your lower back is not rounded and that your tailbone and buttocks do not lift off the floor. If they are, move slightly away. Stretch your legs up, spreading them slightly at hip width. Rest your heels on the wall. Maintain the position and breathe deeply. Keep your arms stretched along your sides, palms on the floor.

Common Mistakes: Bending the knees.

Tips: Breathe deeply while maintaining the position.

RECLINED COW-FACE POSE AT WALL (STRETCHING, FLEXIBILITY, LYING DOWN)

Muscles involved: Stretches the lower body, legs, buttocks, moderate chest opening.

Level: Basic.

Execution: Place the mat near the wall, keeping a pillow handy if needed. Lie on your back, bend your knees at 90 degrees, and place both feet on the wall. Ensure your knees are directly over your hips and your feet are pressed against the wall. Ankles should be aligned with the knees. Place a pillow under your neck for necessary head support. Inhale and try to flatten your spine on the mat. Draw your navel toward your spine and contract your abdominals so there is no arch or space in your lower back. Exhale, bring your feet together. Lift your right foot off the wall. Engage your core and place your right knee over your left knee. Interlace your fingers and wrap them around your left knee. Do not lift your neck. Breathe normally and remain in the pose as long as you can.

To release the pose, unclasp your intertwined fingers and release your crossed legs. Return your feet to the wall as at the start. Repeat the pose on the other side.

Common Mistakes: Holding your breath, arching the lower back.

Tips: Initially, you can simply place your right calf on your left thigh instead of stacking the knees. With practice, you will gain enough flexibility to stack the knees over each other.

22. WORKOUT PLAN

In the guide, you will find 4 types of weekly training plans:

- **Week #1: Beginner Program**

- **Week #2: Program for Improving Flexibility and Balance**

- **Week #3: Weight Loss Program**

- **Week #4: Stress Relief and Back Pain Relief Program**

Each training program is weekly and includes a daily exercise plan for 7 days, totaling 28 days of training.

As you can see, each weekly program has its own specific goal. Within each week, every day focuses on a specific additional goal:

- **Day 1: Let's get started!**

- **Day 2: Full mobility!**

- **Day 3: Full flexibility!**

- **Day 4: Feel your 'core'**

- **Day 5: Stability and balance**

- **Day 6: Flat stomach and toned buttocks**

- **Day 7: Train and Stretch**

This approach ensures a gradual progression both daily and weekly. You'll find some exercises repeated more than others within a week, allowing you to vary the workout while simultaneously gaining familiarity with the exercises.

If you wish to change the order of the weeks or days, you are free to do so. However, I recommend performing the program as proposed, since the degree of difficulty gradually increases day by day, and this will allow you to become familiar with the exercises progressively.

If you want to change the order of execution of the weeks, you can do so, but I suggest starting with the beginner week.

If you find an exercise too difficult or unsuitable, feel free to skip it, but it's important never to skip the initial warm-up and final stretch.

When performing several repetitions of the same exercise, reach your limit. You should not overdo it, but also not be too mild. In the training programs, you will find the number of repetitions or minutes to perform for each exercise. If you reach your limit before the indicated number, stop.

Listen to your body and the sensations you feel. Go with the flow of the exercises and focus on them. What you will gain is a good mood, relaxation, and a great sense of fulfillment.

At the end of each daily workout, devote 3-4 minutes to deep breathing or practice 5 minutes of meditation. This will help you relax and allow your body to experience a state of stillness and oxygenation. It's an excellent way to finish your routine and feel good about continuing with the rest of your daily activities.

Be kind to yourself; don't demand everything right away. Remember that change to achieve better well-being requires patience, one step at a time.

23. WEEK #1 - BEGINNER PROGRAM

Day 1: Let's get started!

1. Standing Alternate Arm Extensions (8-10 reps. per side)...p.37
2. Standing Leg Lateral Swing (8-10 reps. per leg)...p.40
3. Touch Shoulder to Wall (20 reps.)...p.73
4. Alternate Donkey Kick (20 reps.)...p.62
5. Knee Raise with Wall Support (20 reps.)...p.53
6. Push Back to the Wall (8-10 reps.)...p.54
7. Wall Squat (8-10 reps.)...p.63
8. Standing Leg Lateral Thrust (8-10 reps. per leg)...p.76
9. Standing Knee Lift (8-10 reps. per leg)...p.81
10. Face-Down Dog Pose (a couple of min.)...p.82

Day 2: Full mobility!

1. Standing Side Bends (8-10 reps. per side)...p.38
2. Standing Leg Swing (8-10 reps per leg)...p.39
3. Alternate Donkey Kick (20 reps.) ...p.62
4. Standing Simplified Angel to the Wall (8-10 reps.)...p.41
5. Knee Raise with Wall Support (20 reps.) ...p.53
6. Push Back to the Wall (8-10 reps.) ...p.54
7. Leg Circles (8-10 reps. per leg)...p.75
8. Standing Scapular Retraction and Protraction (8-10 reps.)...p.42
9. Standing Knee Lift (8-10 reps. per leg) ...p.81
10. Face-Down Dog Pose (a couple of min.) ...p.82

Day 3: Full flexibility!

1. Standing Alternate Arm Extensions (8-10 reps.)...p.37

2. Standing Lateral Leg Swing (8-10 reps. per leg) …p.40

3. Touch Shoulder to Wall (20 reps.) …p.73

4. Seated Chest Rotation (8-10 reps.)…p.57

5. Seated Touch Toes (8-10 reps. per leg)…p.85

6. Active Frog Stretch (10 reps.)…p.84

7. Bird-Dog Pose with Wall Support (8-10 reps. per side)…p.78

8. Crossing Legs Lying Down (2-3 min.)…p.87

Day 4: Feel your 'core'

1. Standing Side Bends (8 - 10 reps. per side) …p.38

2. Standing Leg Swing (8-10 reps per leg) …p.39

3. Mountain Climber (1-2 min.)…p.55

4. Standing Side Crunches (8-10 reps. per side)…p.77

5. Push Back to the Wall (8-10 reps.) …p.54

6. Wall Squat (8-10 reps.) …p.63

7. Bird-Dog Pose with Wall Support (8-10 reps. per side) …p.78

8. Crossing Legs Lying Down (2-3 min.) …p.87

Day 5: Stability and balance

1. Standing Alternate Arm Extensions (8-10 reps.) …p.37

2. Standing Lateral Leg Swing (8-10 reps. per leg) …p.40

3. Standing Simplified Angel to the Wall (8-10 reps.) …p.41

4. Standing Side Crunches (8-10 reps. per side) …p.77

5. Standing Alternating Shoulder-Arm Circles (20 reps.)…p.44

6. Leg Lateral Thrust (8-10 reps. per leg)…p.76

7. Standing Knee Lift (8-10 reps. per leg) …p.81

8. Face-Down Dog Pose (a couple of min.) …p.82

Day 6: Flat stomach and toned buttocks

1. Standing Side Bends (8 - 10 reps. per side) ...p.38

2. Standing Leg Swing (8-10 reps per leg) ...p.39

3. Mountain Climber (1-2 min.) ...p.55

4. Alternate Donkey Kick (20 reps.) ...p.62

5. Knee Raise with Wall Support (20 reps.) ...p.53

6. Wall Squat (8-10 reps.) ...p.63

7. Semi Lunge with Wall Support (8 - 10 reps. per side)...p.70

8. Elevated Bridge (8-10 reps.)...p.71

9. Crossing Legs Lying Down (2-3 min.) ...p.87

Day 7: Train and Stretch

1. Standing Alternate Arm Extensions (8-10 reps.) ...p.37

2. Standing Lateral Leg Swing (8-10 reps. per leg) ...p.40

3. Kick-Box with Wall Support (20 reps.)...p.52

4. Standing Simplified Angel to the Wall (8-10 reps.) ...p.41

5. Bike Crunch (20 reps.)...p.56

6. Push Back to the Wall (8-10 reps.) ...p.54

7. Wall Squat (8-10 reps.) ...p.63

8. Leg Lateral Thrust (8-10 reps. per leg) ...p.76

9. Elevated Bridge (8-10 reps.) ...p.71

10. Crossing Legs Lying Down (2-3 min.) ...p.87

24. WEEK #2 - PROGRAM FOR IMPROVING FLEXIBILITY AND BALANCE

Day 1: Let's get started!

1. Standing Side Bends (8 - 10 reps. per side) ...p.38

2. Standing Lateral Leg Swing (8-10 reps. per leg) ...p.40

3. Angel to the Wall (8-10 reps.)...p.72

4. Bike Crunch (20 reps.) ...p.56

5. Standing Side Crunches (8-10 reps. per side) ...p.77

6. Bird-Dog Pose with Wall Support (8-10 reps. per side) ...p.78

7. Seated Chest Rotation (8-10 reps.)...p.57

8. Lay Down Hip Mobily (8-10 reps. per side)...p.50

9. Lay Down Wall Walking (2 min.)...p.47

10. Crossing Legs Lying Down (2-3 min.) ...p.87

11. Raised Legs Pose with Heels on Wall (2 min.)...p.88

Day 2: Full mobility!

1. Standing Side Bends (8-10 reps. per side) ...p.38

2. Standing Lateral Leg Swing (8-10 reps. per leg) ...p.40

3. Standing Alternating Shoulder-Arm Circles (20 reps.) ...p.44

4. Cobra pose wall (8-10 reps.)...p.83

5. Standing Side Crunches (8-10 reps. per side) ...p.77

6. Chest Opening (10 reps.)...p.49

7. Bird-Dog Pose with Wall Support (8-10 reps. per side) ...p.78

8. Lay Down Wall Walking (2 min.) ...p.47

9. Crossing Legs Lying Down (2-3 min.) ...p.87

10. Raised Legs Pose with Heels on Wall (2 min.) ...p.88

Day 3: Full flexibility!

1. Mountain Climber (1-2 min.) ...p.55

2. Kick-Box with Wall Support (20 reps.) ...p.52

3. Standing Alternating Shoulder Rotation (10 reps.)...p.43

4. Leg Circles (8-10 reps. per leg) ...p.75

5. Bike Crunch (20 reps.) ...p.56

6. Standing Side Crunches (8-10 reps. per side) ...p.77

7. Chest Opening (10 reps.) ...p.49

8. Seated Chest Rotation (8-10 reps.) ...p.57

9. Lay Down Hip Mobily (8-10 reps. per side) ...p.50

10. Crossing Legs Lying Down (2-3 min.) ...p.87

Day 4: Feel your 'core'

1. Mountain Climber (1-2 min.) ...p.55

2. Standing Kick-Box with Wall Support (20 reps.) ...p.52

3. Bike Crunch (20 reps.) ...p.56

4. Push Back to The Wall (10 reps.) ...p.54

5. Bird-Dog Pose with Wall Support (8-10 reps. per side) ...p.93

6. Elevated Bridge (8-10 reps.) ...p.71

7. Lay Down Alternate Leg Abduction (20 reps.)...p.51

8. Wall Crunches (10 reps.)...p.59

9. Active Frog Stretch (10 reps.) ...p.84

10. Seated Touch Toes (8-10 reps. per leg) ...p.85

11. Seated side bends (1 min per side)...p.80

Day 5: Stability and balance

1. Standing Alternate Arm Extensions (20 reps.) ...p.37

2. Standing Lateral Leg Swing (8-10 reps. per leg) ...p.40

3. Knee Raise with Wall Support (20 reps.) ...p.53

4. Angel to the Wall (8-10 reps.)...p.72

5. Plank Pose with Wall Support (1-2 min.)...p.66

6. Donkey Kicks and Wall Curl (8-10 reps. per leg)...p.74

7. Standing Side Crunches (8-10 reps. per side) ...p.77

8. Leg Circles (8-10 reps. per leg) ...p.75

9. Bird-Dog Pose with Wall Support (8-10 reps. per side) ...p.78

10. Seated Active Forward Bending (8-10 reps.)...p.45

11. Stretching Legs Apart to The Wall (1-2 min.)...p.86

12. Reclined Cow-Face Pose at The Wall (1-2 min. per side)...p.89

Day 6: Flat stomach and toned buttocks

1. Standing Alternate Arm Extensions (20 reps.) ...p.37

2. Mountain Climber (1-2 min.) ...p.55

3. Knee Raise with Wall Support (20 reps.) ...p.53

4. Leg Lateral Thrust (8-10 reps. per leg) ...p.76

5. Bike Crunch (20 reps.) ...p.56

6. Wall Squat (8-10 reps.) ...p.63

7. Semi Lunge with Wall Support (8 - 10 reps. per side)...p.70

8. Elevated Bridge (8-10 reps.) ...p.71

9. Knee to Chest Crunches (20 reps.)...p.60

10. Lay Down Alternate Leg Abduction (20 reps.) ...p.51

11. Crossing Legs Lying Down (2-3 min.) ...p.87

12. Stretching Legs Apart to The Wall (1-2 min.) ...p.86

Day 7: Train and Stretch

1. Standing Side Bends (8 - 10 reps. per side) ...p.38

2. Knee Raise with Wall Support (20 reps.) ...p.53

3. Pressure Arms to The Wall Palms Forward (1-2 min.)...p.64

4. Pressure Arms to The Wall Palms to the Wall (1-2 min.)...p.65

25. WEEK #3 - WEIGHT LOSS PROGRAM

This weekly program incorporates intermittent training by alternating between one day of high-intensity exercise and one day of rest. This approach results in:

- A more effective acceleration of metabolism;

- A greater number of calories burned;

- The muscle recovery necessary to perform the exercises.

Day 1: Let's get started!

1. Mountain Climber (1-2 min.) ...p.55

2. Kick-Box with Wall Support (20 reps.) ...p.52

3. Standing Alternating Shoulder Rotation (10 reps.) ...p.43

4. Leg Circles (8-10 reps. per leg) ...p.75

5. Wall Sit (1-2 min.)...p.68

6. Semi Lunge with Wall Support (8 - 10 reps. per side)...p.70

7. Seated Knee to Chest (20 reps.)...p.46

8. Wall Crunches (10 reps.) ...p.59

9. Lay Down Alternate Leg Abduction (20 reps.) ...p.51

10. Active Frog Stretch (10 reps.) ...p.84

11. Seated Touch Toes (8-10 reps. per leg) ...p.85

12. Seated side bends (1 min per side) ...p.80

Day 2: REST

Day 3: Full flexibility!

1. Mountain Climber (1-2 min.) ...p.55

2. Kick-Box with Wall Support (20 reps.) ...p.52

3. Standing Alternating Shoulder Rotation (10 reps.) ...p.43

4. Leg Circles (8-10 reps. per leg) ...p.75

5. Standing Scapular Retraction and Protraction (8-10 reps.) ...p.57

6. Semi Lunge with Wall Support (8 - 10 reps. per side)...p.70

7. Wall Push Up (10 reps.)...p.69

8. Squat with Stance Change (10 reps.)...p.67

9. Lay Down Alternate Leg Abduction (20 reps.) ...p.51

10. Active Frog Stretch (10 reps.) ...p.84

11. Seated Touch Toes (8-10 reps. per leg) ...p.85

12. Seated Side Bends (1 min per side) ...p.80

Day 4: REST

Day 5: Flat stomach and toned buttocks

1. Mountain Climber (1-2 min.) ...p.55

2. Kick-Box with Wall Support (20 reps.) ...p.52

3. Standing Lateral Leg Swing (8-10 reps. per leg) ...p.40

4. Wall Sit (1-2 min.) ...p.68

5. Semi Lunge with Wall Support (8 - 10 reps. per side) ...p.70

6. Squat with Stance Change (10 reps.) ...p.67

7. Standing Side Crunches (8-10 reps. per side) ...p.77

8. Plank Pose with Wall Support (1-2 min.) ...p.66

9. Standing Pigeon Pose with Wall Support (1-2 min. per leg)...p.79

10. Elevated Bridge (8-10 reps.) ...p.71

11. Knee to Chest Crunches (20 reps.) ...p.60

12. Stretching Legs Apart to The Wall (1-2 min.) ...p.86

13. Reclined Cow-Face Pose at The Wall (1-2 min. per side) ...p.89

Day 6: REST

Day 7: Train and Stretch

1. Mountain Climber (1-2 min.) ...p.55

26. WEEK #4 - STRESS RELIEF AND BACK PAIN RELIEF PROGRAM

Day 1: Let's get started!

1. Standing Alternate Arm Extensions (20 reps.) ...p.37

2. Standing Lateral Leg Swing (8-10 reps. per leg) ...p.40

3. Standing Alternating Shoulder-Arm Circles (20 reps.) ...p.44

4. Standing Scapular Retraction and Protraction (8-10 reps.) ...p.42

5. Donkey Kicks and Wall Curl (8-10 reps. per leg) ...p.74

6. Cobra pose wall (8-10 reps.) ...p.83

7. Wall Push Up (10 reps.) ...p.69

8. Squat With Stance Change (10 reps.) ...p.67

9. Plank Pose with Wall Support (1-2 min.) ...p.66

10. Standing Pigeon Pose with Wall Support (1-2 min. per leg) ...p.79

11. Standing Cat and Cow (10 reps.)...p.48

12. Seated Active Forward Bending (8-10 reps.) ...p.45

13. Stretching Legs Apart to The Wall (1-2 min.) ...p.86

14. Reclined Cow-Face Pose at The Wall (1-2 min. per side) ...p.89

Day 2: Full mobility!

1. Mountain Climber (1-2 min.) ...p.55

2. Kick-Box with Wall Support (20 reps.) ...p.52

3. Standing Alternating Shoulder Rotation (10 reps.) ...p.43

4. Seated Chest Opening (10 reps.) ...p.54

5. Standing Lateral Leg Swing (8-10 reps. per leg) ...p.40

6. Wall Sit (1-2 min.) ...p.68

7. Knee to Chest Crunches (20 reps.) ...p.60

8. Seated Active Forward Bending (8-10 reps.) ...p.45

Day 3: Full flexibility!

Day 4: Feel your 'core'

Day 5: Stability and balance

Day 6: Flat stomach and toned buttocks

6. Pressure Arms to the Wall Palms Forward (1-2 min.)...p.64

7. Pressure Arms to the Wall Palms Against the Wall (1-2 min.)...p.65

8. Knee To Chest Crunches (20 reps.) ...p.60

9. Elevated Bridge (8-10 reps.) ...p.71

10. Crunch with Stretch (10 reps)...p.61

11. Active Frog Stretch (10 reps.) ...p.84

12. Bird-Dog Pose with Wall Support (8-10 reps. per side) ...p.78

13. Alternating Crunch with Wall Support (10 reps)...p.58

14. Stretching Legs Apart to The Wall (1-2 min.) ...p.86

15. Reclined Cow-Face Pose at Wall (1-2 min. per side) ...p.89

Day 7: Train and Stretch

1. Standing Alternate Arm Extensions (20 reps.) ...p.37

2. Standing Lateral Leg Swing (8-10 reps. per leg) ...p.40

3. Standing Alternating Shoulder-Arm Circles (20 reps.) ...p.44

4. Standing Scapular Retraction and Protraction (8-10 reps.) ...p.42

5. Donkey Kicks and Wall Curl (8-10 reps. per leg) ...p.74

6. Cobra Pose (8-10 reps.) ...p.83

7. Wall Push Up (10 reps.) ...p.69

8. Squat with Stance Change (10 reps.) ...p.67

9. Plank Pose with Wall Support (1-2 min.) ...p.66

10. Standing Pigeon Pose with Wall Support (1-2 min. per leg) ...p.79

11. Standing Cat and Cow (10 reps.) ...p.48

12. Seated Active Forward Bending (8-10 reps.) ...p.45

13. Stretching Legs Apart to The Wall (1-2 min.) ...p.86

14. Reclined Cow-Face Pose at Wall (1-2 min. per side) ...p.89

DOWNLOAD YOUR VIDEO WORKOUT PLAN

Finally, you can follow day by day your lessons of

"WALL PILATES WORKOUTS FOR WOMEN" 4 TRAININGS PROGRAMS VIDEOCOURSES.

Practicing your 28-day wall Pilates workout has never been easier. Go to the last page, scan the QR code and gain instant access to:

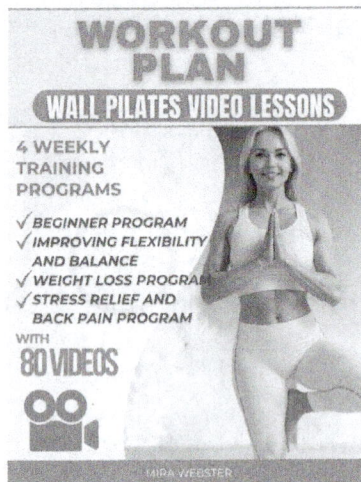

- **WALL PILATES VIDEO WORKOUTS PLAN** -4 weekly programs, featuring 25 video lessons performed by a qualified fitness instructor;

Printed in Dunstable, United Kingdom